D1599112

Hormone Use in
Menopause & Male Andropause

Hormone Use in
Menopause & Male Andropause

· · · · · · ·

A Choice for Women and Men

Sheldon J. Segal, Ph.D. & Luigi Mastroianni, Jr., M.D.

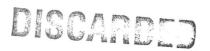

OXFORD
UNIVERSITY PRESS

2003

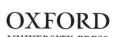

OXFORD
UNIVERSITY PRESS

Oxford   New York
Auckland   Bangkok   Buenos Aires   Cape Town   Chennai
Dar es Salaam   Delhi   Hong Kong   Istanbul   Karachi   Kolkata
Kuala Lumpur   Madrid   Melbourne   Mexico City   Mumbai   Nairobi
São Paulo   Shanghai   Taipei   Tokyo   Toronto

Library of Congress Cataloging-in-Publication Data
Segal, Sheldon J. (Sheldon Jerome)
Hormone use in menopause and male andropause : a choice
for women and men / by Sheldon J. Segal & Luigi Mastroianni, Jr.
p. ; cm.
Includes bibliographical references and index.
ISBN 0-19-515974-8
1. Menopause.   2. Middle aged women—Health and hygiene.
3. Climacteric, Male.   4. Middle aged men—Health and hygiene.
5. Climacteric.
[DNLM: 1. Climacteric—physiology—Popular Works.
2. Menopause—physiology—Popular Works.   3. Hormone Replacement
Therapy—Popular Works. WP 580 S454n 2003]   I. Mastroianni, Luigi.
II. Title.
RG186.S43 2003
612.6'65—dc21   2002154499

9 8 7 6 5 4 3 2 1

Printed in the United States of America
on acid-free paper

For **HARRIET** and **ELAINE**

• • • Preface

We decided to write this book to help women and men find their way through the maze of information, sometimes conflicting, about one of the important issues in their lives: How to handle the bodily changes brought on in the post-reproductive years. For women the phrase "post-reproductive years" is very literal. Aging brings a clear dividing line between the time that a woman is biologically capable of reproducing and the time that she is not. Men may retain the biological ability to reproduce well into an advanced age but, practically speaking, their reproductive years usually correspond to those of women. We believed that one book that addressed the questions raised by changes accompanying aging in women as well as those changes in men would be helpful. After all, couples age together. A visitor from Mars, browsing in the health section of a Barnes & Noble store, might come to the conclusion that on Earth only women grow older!

You don't have to be a demographer to know that women now spend about a third of their lives in the postmenopausal years, and as life expectancy increases, the added years are menopausal. Males reach their biological peak before they are twenty, you hear, and then it is all downhill. That's a distortion of facts, but it is true that testosterone production in men starts to decline fairly early in life. The growing use of testosterone products by older men shows that they don't want to take this passively. Like women who have flocked to hormone therapy for menopause, aging men, hoping to improve the quality of their lives, want a piece of the hormone action.

We are both academic endocrinologists, one with a lifetime experience as a practicing obstetrician/gynecologist and the other as a research scientist who has had a productive career studying reproductive hormones and their mechanisms of action. We have collaborated on scientific projects and worked together in the activities of our professional societies. Early in our careers, we moved into our first departmental chairmanships the same year, and were elected together to the U.S. National Academy of Sciences Institute of Medicine. But the experience that convinced us that we could work together to produce a co-authored book is the sharing of a sailboat. That's the true test of compatibility. Not unimportantly, it gave us the opportunity to spend countless hours on the changing waters of Vineyard Sound off Cape Cod, Massachusetts, talking about our work and exchanging views. We decided that sharing our thoughts and opinions with the general public could be a service and were pleased when Oxford University Press agreed to publish our book and that we were able to work with Kirk Jensen, our excellent editor.

From the start, we agreed that the hallmark of our book would be evidence-based medicine and science. In a field where there is considerable anecdotal information and unsubstantiated claims, we believed it would be important to base our writings and recommendations on publications in the scientific and medical literature. All told, we use information from nearly 500 articles that we list in the back of the book for those who might want to go to the original sources for more details.

We have organized the book into three parts. The first two parts cover questions we are asked about menopause (part I) and andropause (part II), respectively. These questions are dealt with in some detail, but we try to avoid the jargon that is part of our professions. Part III is a compilation of short answers to the questions that we and our professional colleagues are asked by patients and others who seek our opinions and advice. The commentary provides an overview of the important Women's Health Initiative (WHI) study that received worldwide publicity in 2002.

Our work on andropause had a similar encounter with timely news. Shortly after the WHI news flurry, reporters learned that the National Institutes of Health decided not to fund a similar long-term study on the risks and benefits of the male version of hormone replacement therapy because it would be difficult to carry to completion and would cost more than $100 million. We share the disappointment of many of our colleagues that this proposed study did not go forward, but this does not mean that there is a dearth of scientific publications on andropause, which we share with you in this book.

We gratefully acknowledge the help, advice, and criticism generously offered by our colleagues and friends. L. M. Jr. expresses his gratitude to his colleagues of the Department of Obstetrics and Gynecology of the University of Pennsylvania School of Medicine and, in particular, to Celso-Ramon Garcia and to his long-time administrative assistant Valerie Baldwin. S.J.S. thanks the many people with whom he interacted and exchanged views while working on the book at the Rockefeller Foundation's Study and Conference Center, Bellagio, Italy. In particular, he extends thanks for the valuable suggestions he received while in Bellagio from Larry Tye, Jean-Pierre Habicht, and Regine Sitruk-Ware. He also acknowledges with admiration the critiques offered by Professor of Urology Julian Frick of Innsbruck, Austria.

The wisdom and suggestions we have received from these colleagues have been invaluable to assure accuracy but any errors that remain are our own.

• • • Commentary: The Women's Health Initiative Clinical Study

As this book was nearing completion, the *Journal of the American Medical Association* (JAMA) published an article that dramatically reshaped public attitudes toward hormone therapy for women in menopause. It reported interim results of the U.S. National Institutes of Health (NIH) Women's Health Initiative, the largest-ever study of its kind, which was launched in 1993 and was scheduled to be completed in 2005. The abrupt termination of a critical part of the study generated such sweeping and often misleading headlines that we felt compelled to add this special commentary to a book that already addresses all the substantive issues raised by the NIH study.

In the Women's Health Initiative (WHI) clinical trial thousands of women around the country were placed on a popular hormone therapy (HT), while thousands of others were given placebo pills. The intent was simple: to measure whether the benefits of HT outweigh the risks. The plan was that if the benefits proved obvious midway, this part of the study would be stopped so women on the placebo could switch to hormone therapy. Conversely, if dangers became apparent, the study would be stopped early to prevent additional risks.

It is not surprising that the abrupt halting of the study would be considered newsworthy. The message, however, has been distorted. The $170 million trial was ended because a statistical trigger was reached that led the NIH evaluating committee to conclude that the overall health risks exceeded the benefits and it would be unnecessary to continue women on medication for three more years. But while they had reached a predetermined criterion for stopping the study, they had not arrived at an answer to the critical question of risks versus benefits.

The primary reason for calling an early end to this phase of the NIH study was a concern that Prempro, the most widely used hormone therapy and the one researchers zeroed in on, causes a worrisome increase in adverse events including breast cancer and cardiac disease. But when you cut through the statistical corrections, boundaries, and indices underlying the decision to terminate the study, the absolute excess risk of major adverse events was 19 per 10,000 women-years of use. After an average of 5.2 years of observation, absolute excess risks per 10,000 women per year of use attributable to Prempro were 7 more heart disease events, 8 more strokes, 8 more pulmonary embolisms, and 8 more diagnosed breast cancers. Absolute risk reductions per 10,000 women per year of use were 6 fewer colorectal cancers and 5 fewer hip fractures. There also were fewer vertebral and other bone fractures, although those were not included in the calculation of benefit increases, and other cases of thrombosis were not counted.

Bottom line: The reduction in colorectal cancers almost cancelled out the increase in breast cancer, and a change in just a few cases in any of the adverse events categories could have shifted the risk/benefit analysis. That's how small the measure of difference was between the two groups. The shift would have been even greater if the alleviation of menopause symptoms had been factored into the results as beneficial. And there was no difference in mortality rates between the two groups.

The second concern we have about the study's termination—and the way it has been interpreted—is that the Women's Health Initiative clinical trial never really represented the population for whom hormone therapy makes most sense. Women with extreme symptoms of menopause were excluded since they would continue to suffer those symptoms if they were randomly assigned to the placebo group and did not receive any treatment. That would be unethical. However, these are precisely the women for whom most prescriptions for hormone therapy are written. Eighty-five percent of prescriptions for Prempro and similar products are for less-than-five-year users who are taking HT for quality of life complaints. This exclusion criterion eliminated from the study many women just entering menopause so that the average age of the study group, at 63.2 years, was far older than newly menopausal women in general. That also means that the preexistence of other diseases of aging, including early stages of atherosclerosis, was hard to exclude. About one-third of the women in the study were being treated for hypertension and 69% were overweight. Preexisting heart disease or diabetes was reported by 13% of the women. In other words, the project studied a small subsection of hormone therapy users, and the adverse events were concentrated in an even smaller subsection.

As the study progressed, there were other pragmatic reasons guided by good clinical care of the women that resulted in further dilution of the intended chance assignment. Some experts in study design believe that it is not possible to achieve true random assignment in an ethical clinical trial. The pitfalls of this study might prove it.

There are several other worries we have about the way the NIH trial was terminated. For one, the added risk of breast cancer was what triggered stopping the trial. Yet, the breast cancers detected probably were not new tumors but were preexisting ones brought up to detectable size by the hormone stimulation, which actually could ensure they are detected and treated. And even with that caveat, the 6% rate of increase in diagnosis of breast cancer among study subjects who were getting their first HT treatment was statistically insignificant, meaning that it could be purely a matter of chance.

What disturbs us most, however, is that after the press got an early look at the JAMA article, reports tended to overstate the cautionary findings and emphasize the abrupt halt. In response, anxious women began contacting their doctors, some abandoned their prescribed medication, editorials were written, and litigation lawyers started advertising for clients. Yet it took over a week for doctors to get their paper copies of JAMA, at which point they could closely scrutinize the actual findings, recognize that there was no cause for panic, and reassure anxious patients. The study had stopped but this did not mean that women needed to stop using hormone therapy.

Reports based on information gathered in the WHI study have continued to come out. Almost every report is counterintuitive and contradicts the findings of literally hundreds of previous studies in the scientific literature. An analysis of WHI records published by JAMA in March 2003 concludes that HT does no better than a placebo in reducing most menopausal symptoms. However, this is contrary to the experience reported by millions of American women who started to use hormones as they began to have menopausal complaints. A closer look at the WHI information may explain this paradox. The study excluded women with extreme symptoms of menopause, so it cannot tell us how the treatment works for women experiencing debilitating problems with hot flashes and night sweats. Perhaps on this issue all the study proves is that if a woman is trouble-free to begin with, hormone therapy cannot make her more trouble-free.

In June 2003, two more papers appeared in JAMA describing how older women (age 65–70) in the WHI study performed in various psychological tests measuring cognitive skills. Previous evidence from many studies indicated that HT can *improve* cognitive function and *delay* the onset of Alzheimer's disease. Yet the WHI found that for some women HT can *increase* the risk of dementia. This is the news item that found its way into press headlines. Most troubling and enigmatic was a follow-up report on breast cancer, also in June 2003, concluding that estrogen plus progestin may not only stimulate growth of cancer cells, but may also hinder breast cancer diagnosis by mammography. The enigma is that in the decades of growing use of both HT and mammography by American women, breast cancer mortality rates have steadily declined.

Professionals providing health care and the women who seek their counsel are faced with a dilemma. On the one hand, they can succumb to the notion, fueled by reports in the lay press, that the results of a single randomized, placebo controlled study supercedes the information assembled from a large number of studies based on animal experiments, labortory results, sophisticated diagnostic measures, neurological evaluations, clinical trials involving human subjects, and epidemiological evidence. Or, at some point, they may question that perhaps the WHI study's design or implementation has fundamental imperfections. Are the subjects actually representative of typical postmenopausal women, or have the study's criteria for inclusion and exclusion inadvertently selected out a nonrepresentative subgroup of women? Does the elevated average age of subjects in the WHI (63 years) influence the study's outcome? The study's sponsors report that the results are consistent across all age subgroups but this dissection of the total shrinks the numbers being compared considerably. With the overall net total of 19 adverse events per 10,000 women-years of use, the numbers of events in the age subgroups must be in the single digits. Another puzzling element is the high dropout rate. A substantial number of women (42%) stopped taking study drugs at some time during the WHI study.

We think the Women's Health Initiative study has revealed important information but it also has limitations. It is not at all clear to us that the study has provided the final word on issues that are so important to women entering menopause or to women who have been using hormone therapy to control menopausal symptoms. An objective and careful appraisal of the WHI is needed, to try to understand why the study's conclusions differ so widely from the results of a large body of reputable scientific evidence. This is not our purpose in this book but we hope that the comprehensive information from the overall medical and scientific literature that we present here will help set the record straight.

• • • Contents

Part III • Questions and Answers

1 • • • Menopause

1 • Why do women have menopause?

Menopause is the result of an inevitable decline in ovarian function. The term usually denotes the completion of a full year without a menstrual period. As menopause approaches, the ovaries decrease in size as virtually all the egg-containing ovarian follicles are lost due to a process called atresia. Estrogen production diminishes, and cycles tend to become shorter and more erratic. Menopause follows this last phase of the life cycle of the ovary which starts early in fetal life when the gland mobilizes the resources it will later need to assure egg and hormone production throughout a woman's reproductive years.

The link between deterioration of ovarian function and menopause is the fall in estrogen production. Estrogen is not only important for maintaining reproductive function, but it is a key hormone in maintaining bone density and for protecting against other physical and mental health disorders associated with aging. Sleep disturbances, hot flashes, vaginal dryness, and urinary incontinence are all conditions associated with estrogen fluctuation or deprivation. Osteoporosis, thinning of the bones, is a life-threatening condition for postmenopausal women. The onset of menopause, in other words, has many more health-related implications for women than simply the loss of reproductive capacity.

The average age of menopause in the United States is 51.4 years, but the range that is considered normal is wide—from age 42 to age 58. Since American women now live, on the average, to age 80, they spend more than a third of their lives in the postmenopausal phase. As women's life expectancy increases (and it is projected to rise to 82 by 2025), the years added will be allotted to life beyond the onset of menopause.

For the human female, ovarian differentiation is a defining moment of lifelong consequence. That immature gland will emerge as the controlling factor for many crucial features of her life, in addition to providing her with the fertility that will enable her to bear children. The ovary will determine when she reaches puberty and starts to menstruate. It will control the regularity of her periods and the symptoms that she may have to live with month after month during her reproductive years. The ovary's demise will determine when she will no longer menstruate and thus enter menopause.

The inevitability of a woman's menopause is linked to the life history of her ovary. It is a sequence of events followed in every woman under normal circumstances and one that has been unchanged since the evolution of our species. The story begins with the determination of sex at fertilization when the chromosomes of the egg and sperm are paired. Since eggs normally carry a single X chromosome, if the fertilizing sperm carries a male sex chromosome (Y chromosome), the makeup becomes XY, and the newly fertilized egg is destined to develop into a male. The fusion of an X-bearing sperm with an egg results in a female chromosomal constitution (XX) which will guide the development of ovaries.

For several weeks after fertilization, as development begins, the chromosomal constitution is the only distinguishing feature between male and female fertilized eggs or early embryos. To discover which genetic sex was established at fertilization, you would somehow have to capture the developing embryo as it makes its journey from the upper end of the Fallopian tube, the usual arena of fertilization, through the tortuous turns of the tube, past the tubal-uterine junction and into the uterine cavity. After finding the embryo, you would need to do a sex chromosome analysis or DNA fingerprinting. The impracticality of this is obvious. Even after the embryo begins to implant in the lining of the uterus at about day six to seven after fertilization, nothing about it other than the encoded sex chromosomes can reveal the difference between a male and female. This uniform appearance prevails for several weeks as the early stages of embryo development unfold.

The first physical difference appears when the gonads differentiate as either ovaries or testes. Along a fold of a supportive membrane in the abdomen, near the developing kidney, a ridge, referred to as the gonadal ridge, starts to thicken where the future gonad (testis or ovary) will appear.

Nothing further happens until migrating cells from a distant location arrive and take up residence. This triggers the start of gonad development. At this point, the first physical difference between males and females begins to take shape. If the embryo is female, migrating stem cells tend to aggregate in the outer cell layers of the gonadal ridge. In the nascent ovary, these primitive stem cells, together with support cells they acquire along their route, form simple follicles, the structures that will eventually contain eggs and produce reproductive hormones. The ovarian follicles are destined, after puberty, to give rise to the woman's main source of estrogen. As long as the ovaries contain follicles, they will produce the eggs and the hormones that define the reproductive phase of a woman's life.

If the embryo is male and the gonad is to be a testis, convoluted tubules form the structures that house the stem cells that will ultimately give rise to sperm. Different cells that are formed outside of the tubes will produce testosterone. The anatomical separation of cells that produce sperm and cells that produce hormones is important for the testes' future history.

The embryonic ovary is initially populated by just a handful of primitive stem cells, sheathed in their rudimentary follicles. These cells (oogonia) will eventually give rise to eggs. The oogonia rapidly multiply so that during fetal life their numbers grow astronomically. Millions of these potential egg cells are found in each ovary at the height of this multiplication phase of ovarian development at about the sixth month of pregnancy.

Why this abundance is necessary has never been understood, for no sooner does this cell population explosion take place than the potential egg cells begin to degenerate. This degenerative process, referred to as atresia, dominates ovarian activity throughout the remainder of fetal life and continues thereafter, ultimately claiming 99.99% of the cells having the potential to become eggs. However, human reproduction is successful, and the species survives because some of the oogonia stop dividing and enter into a maturation process to become a more advanced cell type (oocyte), capable of becoming mature fertilizable eggs. By birth, the ovary contains about a million oocytes, each encapsulated in a primary follicle. Atresia has caused the destruction of all the rest of the many millions of oogonia that had the potential to become eggs. During the years of childhood and preadolescence, the atresia process continues, reducing the number of oocytes in the young ovaries even further. The follicle count falls to less than half a million as puberty approaches. The cell counts mentioned are estimates based on sparse information but indicate the order of magnitude of follicle distribution at different stages of ovarian development.

The average age of puberty, when the ovary emerges from its long period of inactivity, is about 12 years. It can occur earlier. I've had the sad experience of delivering a baby to a nine-year-old, a victim of incestual rape, barely old enough to understand what was happening to her.

As puberty (menarche) approaches, usually there is an erratic period of irregular cycles, some ovulatory, some anovulatory, before the more or less normal periodicity of ovulation and menstruation becomes established. This is what the ovary prepared for many years earlier when the multiplication phase came to an end and oocyte maturation and follicle development began. Along with this awakening of ovarian function, the atresia process persists, so that for every egg that is released at midcycle, countless others degenerate, maintaining the relentless depopulation of the ovaries.

Ovulation itself, vital for the species' survival, plays a miniscule role in this process. In a woman's lifetime, a few hundred eggs, at most, are released. Consider that the average age of puberty is 12 years and the age of menopause is 51 among American women. Hypothetically, this means 39 years of 13 menstrual cycles a year, or potentially 500 eggs released at ovulation. But the average American woman will have two pregnancies and will breast-feed about 28 weeks after each pregnancy. This natural ovulation suppression eliminates approximately 50 ovulations, and since there are frequent anovulatory cycles around puberty and as menopause approaches, the actual number of eggs released in a woman's lifetime is probably no more than 400—a statistically insignificant number compared to the millions present in the fetal ovary or the hundreds of thousands present at puberty.

The inexorable emptying of the ovaries of oocytes and their surrounding follicle cells causes the deterioration of ovarian function and carries a woman to menopause. When there is no longer an adequate supply of follicles in the ovary, the hormonal cycles associated with ovulation cease, and the reproductive phase of a woman's life comes to an end. Atresia, not ovulation, is the controlling factor in this process. Even if every ovulation a woman can have were somehow prevented, it would contribute little to the ultimate depletion of the ovary's egg and follicle supply. Taking the ovulation-suppressing oral contraceptive pill, for example, from puberty onward would not affect the age of menopause significantly. Actually, nature has done that experiment for us throughout history. Throughout history when women were either pregnant or breast-feeding for most of their reproductive years, they rarely ovulated. Yet, anthropological evidence suggests that for surviving women the average age of menopause was the same as it is today.

What might delay menopause would be a pill that not only stops ovulation but also stops atresia, so that even with advancing years, the ovary would remain richly endowed with follicles and monthly ovulations and menstruations would be possible. There is no such pill (or other form of medication.) For women, aging will bring on menopause, as surely as will surgical removal of both ovaries at any time in adult life. Menopause is built into a woman's genetic makeup. It is inevitable.

We cannot be certain that the only factor responsible for menopause is depletion of follicles within the ovary. The pituitary gland and the brain's hypothalamus, which controls the pituitary gland, are key players in the endocrinology of reproduction and may have a built-in senescence. Molecular biologists have identified several genes that influence atresia, but this confirms that the process is complex and not amenable to simple explanations. Genes that control the depletion of ovarian follicles in the fetus may be different from those controlling atresia in the adult ovary.

Throughout the reproductive years, in response to hormonal signals from the hypothalamus and pituitary, each month a woman's estrogen production follows a pattern that is defined by her ovulatory cycle. During the first half of the month, a cluster of primary follicles start to develop, and their cells produce estrogen that is released into the bloodstream. Early in this follicular phase of the cycle, one dominant follicle takes over and the others deteriorate and disappear. The blood level of estrogen, primarily estradiol, rises to a peak at about mid-cycle. This triggers other hormonal events that result in ovulation and a precipitous drop in estrogen production as the vacated follicle shifts to producing progesterone as the main hormone for the second half of the cycle. Estrogen production, however, never declines to zero and, in fact, has a second peak during the progesterone-dominated phase, as a new crop of follicles is mobilized and begins developing for the next cycle in case a pregnancy does not take place.

This process continues month after month, year after year, as long as a fertile woman has an adequate supply of follicles. The intervention of a pregnancy does not deprive a woman of estrogen, for the levels are high as the placenta takes over the function of producing estrogen while the ovary is taking a pregnancy-induced time out. This is why women can retain their estrogen-stimulated characteristics and health parameters whether they have one baby in their lifetime or eight, as was the average fertility rate in the days of colonial America.

The physiological basis of menopause is the estrogen decline resulting from depletion of ovarian follicles. Although it is axiomatic that follicle numbers decline with aging, it is not possible to verify this with observational data because follicle counts correlated with age are rare and are derived using crude counting methods. Mathematical modeling based on the limited information available predicts that in normal women follicle depletion accelerates after the age of 38. This is when estrogen levels in the blood (averaged over a month) begin a steep decline. Yet, robust ovarian function and successful fertility can be maintained for many years beyond this threshold.

The decline and cessation of ovarian function are programmed into every woman's biological clock. This is menopause. Predicting its onset for an individual woman is a challenge that modern science has not yet been able to meet.

2 • What are the signs of menopause?

At some point in a woman's life she will experience bodily changes that herald the onset of the menopause. Hot flashes, sleeplessness, night sweats, and mood swings are the most familiar signs, but there are many other significant changes as a woman enters a new phase of life. This period of life is frequently called "perimenopause." It is usually defined as the years leading up to menopause and includes up to one year after the final menses.

The complaint that usually prompts the first perimenopausal visit to the doctor's office is a change in the pattern of menstrual bleeding. Women expect this change and can tell when it is happening. Except for the pathological condition of premature menopause, I cannot recall an instance of a patient registering surprise when I confirmed that the symptoms that brought her to my office were the first signs of menopause.

Many women are aware of subtle changes in body composition. They are particularly concerned about a tendency to gain weight because of fat deposition around the hips and abdomen. With just a glance in a full-length mirror, a perimenopausal woman is aware that her body shape is changing.

The changes a woman feels at this time of life are the result of increasing deviations from the pattern of hormonal changes characteristic of the normal menstrual cycle. Diminishing ovarian function is the main reason for this alteration. This is part of the normal lifetime physiology of a woman's body. It is part of her genetic makeup. Ovulation is less frequent and more irregular, and the ovary produces estrogen in sporadic and unpredictable amounts. This is because the neat feedback system that allows the pituitary gland to monitor and regulate physiological function breaks down.

The corpus luteum, the structure normally formed from the vacated follicle after an egg is released from the ovary, is not present if there has been no ovulation. Consequently, the progesterone-dominated phase of the cycle is absent, and orderly growth of the uterine lining followed by a controlled menstrual flow does not occur. Without progesterone, the pituitary gland does not get the proper signals to keep everything going smoothly as in the usual menstrual cycle. The endometrium, or uterine lining, is subjected to erratic stimulation by estrogen alone, and the woman's bleeding pattern becomes irregular. Women begin to experience either absence of periods or extended intervals between periods. There can be an abrupt halt to menstrual cycles and, for many women, menstruation never resumes.

Another pattern of change is characterized by unexplained, excessive menstrual blood loss. As ovarian function starts to change, stimulation by estrogen alone without the balancing role of progesterone can cause excessive buildup of the endometrium, followed by sloughing. This pattern can be manifested as irregular bleeding which can be simple staining or, in more extreme cases, hemorrhage resulting in significant blood loss. Because it is the result of dysfunctional ovarian function, this irregular menstrual pattern of the perimenopause is known as "dysfunctional uterine bleeding."

In an ovulatory cycle, the menstrual period is of a fixed duration. The amount and duration of flow differs only slightly from one cycle to the next. When the endometrium has been stimulated only by estrogen, breakthrough bleeding can be variable in amount and duration, as described above. Uncontrolled hemorrhage can be extremely serious and requires immediate medical attention. Usually this dysfunctional bleeding responds to the administration of a progestin-containing pill to substitute for the progesterone that would be produced in a normal cycle. When the breakthrough bleeding does not respond to this type of medication, it can be controlled by a large dose of estrogen alone. This causes the endometrium to proliferate, and the ruptured blood vessels responsible for the breakthrough bleeding are repaired. Once the bleeding is under control, progesterone can be added to the treatment for several days, and a relatively normal flow usually ensues. This approach is sometimes referred to as "medical curettage." The objective is to build up and stabilize the endometrium. When the medication is stopped, within a few days there is an organized sloughing of endometrial tissue in the form of a manageable menstrual period.

Not long ago, the treatment of dysfunctional uterine bleeding was an immediate dilation and curettage (D&C) requiring hospitalization and surgery. Some women endured not one but several D&Cs to get through the dysfunctional bleeding phase of menopause. This is no longer standard practice. Now that highly effective progestin agents are available for treatment, the invasive procedure can usually be avoided. Once the acute bleeding phase has been brought under control, it is prudent to have the uterine lining examined by a pathologist. A tissue sample is usually obtained by inserting a small plastic tube past the cervix into the uterine cavity and collecting a sample of the endometrium, which is sent to the pathologist for evaluation.

The marked fluctuations in estrogen level during perimenopause sometimes result in excessive stimulation of the lining cells of the endometrium, resulting in the condition referred to as "hyperplasia." Endometrial hyperplasia simply means increased (hyper-) growth of the endometrium. In extreme cases, the glands of the endometrium become hyperactive, a condition called "adenomatous hyperplasia." Adenomatous hyperplasia is caused by estrogen. Because it can lead to endometrial cancer, carefully monitoring the progression of this condition is essential. Women can reduce the risk of excessive stimulation of the endometrium inherent in estrogen-only hormone replacement regimens by using products that include a progestin in combination with estrogen. This is what physicians prescribe if a woman has not had a hysterectomy and decides to start hormone therapy. This is a benefit of estrogen-plus-progestin hormone therapy that is beyond dispute.

Change in menstrual bleeding pattern, though prominent during perimenopause, is but one of the harbingers of menopause. The array of symptoms can have many different causes. Not all are physiological. They are certainly age related, occurring in concert with other dramatic life changes. Interactions with children, job responsibilities, and marital relationships are often most complicated at this point in a woman's life, but physiological factors should not be underestimated.

Women with a history of symptoms associated with ovulation and menstruation often note that these are accentuated during perimenopause. If a woman has experienced premenstrual syndrome (PMS), those symptoms, too, can be markedly magnified, resulting in increased irritability and a sense of inability to cope with day-to-day situations. Changes in sleeping patterns are often experienced, which aggravates other symptoms. The body is stressed and tired, and yet sleep is elusive. The fluctuating estrogen levels during perimenopause can trigger bursts of night sweats. After finally dozing off, the woman is awakened by a sense of overheating, and the bed sheets may be drenched with perspiration.

These body-temperature–related changes are referred to as the "vasomotor symptoms" of menopause because they are caused by expansion and contraction of blood vessels, processes that are controlled by the nerves supplying the tiny muscular layer of veins and capillaries throughout the body. Vasomotor changes are probably the clearest example of the effect of estrogen deprivation on a woman's body. We know this because menopausal estrogen therapy almost invariably suppresses the vasomotor symptoms within a matter of days.

As mentioned above, the main sign or symptom of menopause is amenorrhea: the absence of the menstrual cycles and periods. Before the actual cessation of menses, symptoms may occur in spurts, followed by intervals of normalcy. For some women, normal ovulatory menstrual cycles can return for a while, followed by a reappearance of menopausal symptoms. Patients may stop ovulating for several months and, for reasons that are inexplicable, once again begin to ovulate and menstruate normally. If menstrual cramps were part of the pattern in the past, these symptoms return, as cramping is typically associated with an ovulatory menstrual cycle and not with one in which ovulation does not occur (anovulatory cycle). This is because without the vacated follicle, or corpus luteum, after ovulation there is no progesterone-stimulated build up of the uterine lining, which ultimately leads to a production of prostaglandin, the cramp-causing hormone. Prostaglandin inhibitors such as aspirin provide relief of menstrual cramps (dysmenorrhea) for this reason.

Because of the effect of aging on the eggs, fertility is not usually restored in these late-onset ovulatory cycles. When so-called menopausal pregnancies do occur, they are associated with a high incidence of miscarriage and, if the pregnancy progresses to the delivery of a newborn, frequent developmental or genetic abnormalities including Down's syndrome.

Genital atrophy including thinning of the vaginal wall and vaginal dryness is an important part of the bodily changes brought on by menopause. Changes in sexual satisfaction and libido often occur. Prevention of genital atrophy can be an important part of helping women adjust to the bodily changes of the menopause. Estrogen treatment can prevent or improve genital atrophy but has minimal effect on libido in most women. The loss of sexual interest and libido may be the result of reduced production of testosterone, a normal hormonal function for premenopausal women. This theory is supported by the anecdotal reports of menopausal women that the inclusion of small amounts of testosterone in hormone therapy can improve sexual function. They find that the addition of testosterone results in significant improvement in sexual desire, satisfaction, and frequency.

Many women, as they pass into menopause, do not experience symptoms of irregular or heavy bleeding. In the majority of cases, there is gradual cessation or even an abrupt halt of ovulation, followed by complete absence of menstruation. In about 10–15% of aging women there are no further symptoms. For other women, menopause is characterized by extreme symptoms such as severe hot flashes which cannot be controlled and which can occur at any time. Hot flashes can be triggered by tension or stressful life situation or sometimes for no apparent reason.

There are also occult signs of menopause that a woman needs to be sure not to neglect. Bone density, for example, should be evaluated. Several classes of drugs that can prevent the loss of bone minerals are now available. As she approaches menopause, a woman should realize that her risks for cardiovascular disease are increased, so she should become more aware of blood lipid patterns. Diet, exercise, and weight control are among the measures that can slow the progression of atherosclerosis, along with many prescription products that can cause a reduction in the body's production of cholesterol.

Urinary incontinence occurs frequently among older women. Any level of incontinence is not only inconvenient and disagreeable but can lead to disability and social isolation. Mechanical factors involving the shift in location of the pelvic organs, rather than hormonal changes, are most likely responsible. This debilitating condition is not an inevitable result of menopause. Both lifestyle choices and therapeutic options are available for prevention and treatment of this condition. Reduction of caffeine intake helps many women, and there are special exercises (Kegel vaginal contractions) designed to strengthen the pelvic floor. There is extensive scientific literature on the value of these exercises. When prevention does not work, the urinary symptoms can be managed with medication, including vaginal or oral estrogen, supportive prosthetic devices, or even surgery.

The signs and symptoms of menopause may be inexorable, but women do not have to live with them. The cessation of ovarian function and the bodily changes brought about by this change may be inevitable, but a woman has many choices for dealing with each of the symptoms that would otherwise interfere with the quality of her life during the menopausal years.

3 • What is menopausal hormone therapy?

The term "hormone replacement therapy" (HRT) probably has a commercial origin but doctors and women accepted it for several decades. That changed after the release of the interim report from the Women's Health Initiative (WHI) study in July 2002. Shortly afterward, the National Institutes of Health recommended that the term "menopausal hormone therapy" would be preferable. The familiar term "hormone replacement therapy" will thus soon become obsolete as the Food and Drug Administration requires pharmaceutical companies to act on this recommendation regarding nomenclature.

Because menopause is brought about by the decrease in levels of ovarian hormones, the initial rationale was that replacing these hormones could offset the deficiency. The term "HRT" implies that the replacement of the diminished natural hormone production prevents the symptoms of estrogen deprivation. "Replacement" would be an acceptable description of the hormone therapy if, indeed, one could determine the precise hormonal status of perimenopausal women and were able to customize treatment for each woman. This is not what usually happens and, in fact, would be very impractical. Efforts have been made to do this hormonal calibration using a simple saliva test. The test has been available for many years but it is not widely used. In most cases, it is no more helpful than having the health care provider determine what may be required on the basis of an examination and the symptoms reported by a patient.

There is no way to decide automatically what therapy is best for each individual; one formula does not fit all. Understandably, this is usually the first question asked by a woman considering the use of hormones for the treatment of menopausal symptoms: What is the best method? There is no simple answer. Most health care providers tend to have a preferred product or dose of hormones that, in their experience, has worked well. What may be appropriate for one woman, however, might prove to be excessive treatment or under dosing in another. Consequently, it is not unusual for the first months of treatment to be a trial-and-error interval to establish the right hormones, mode of delivery, and doses for each woman.

By far, the most widely used treatment contains the conjugated estrogens in Premarin, the first product to be approved by the U.S. Food and Drug Administration (FDA) for indications associated with menopause. Pregnant mare's urine is the source of these water-soluble estrogen conjugates (and thus the derivation of its name). This source of estrogen was discovered by Bernhard Zondek.

Zondek, one of the pioneers in hormone research, was an Israeli doctor the who started his career as a young physician in Germany in the 1920s. This was the dawn of endocrinology, and as the understanding of reproductive hormones began to evolve, Zondek was credited with one new discovery after another. He was so actively involved in research on the hormones of pregnancy that he was sometimes introduced, tongue in cheek, as the man who invented pregnancy. With the rise of Nazism, Zondek fled to Jerusalem and escaped the Holocaust.

Zondek was an inveterate storyteller. I enjoyed listening to tales of his early work that ultimately led to the first FDA-approved menopausal hormone therapy. Zondek discovered that the pregnant mare produces bountiful amounts of estrogen in conjugated form that can be found in the ovaries, blood, or urine of the mare during pregnancy. He told me of his surprise when, as a young man from Berlin, he came to Paris to present a lecture on this subject and was greeted at the hotel by a group who introduced themselves as businessmen who had started a company to produce equine estrogens for human use, based on Zondek's discovery. He accepted their offer of a fine dinner, the only pecuniary reward he ever received for his discovery, and a visit to the farm-factory outside Paris where pregnant mare urine was being collected for extraction of the hormones. There, he saw a sturdy, well-fed stallion presiding over row after row of pregnant mares, each in a stall connected to an elaborate piping system that funneled their urine to a central vat where the isolation of the hormones could begin. While he watched, dazzled by the sophistication of the operation, someone called, "Bernhard!" He turned toward the voice, startled that someone he hardly knew would address him by his first name, and noticed that the stallion turned, also. Proudly, his hosts explained, "We named him after you!"

Many years later and after countless additional scientific studies on the subject, Zondek's discovery became the basis for the family of Premarin products, the most widely used prescription drug ever marketed for women's health. Premarin products became a $2 billion a year industry and still dominate the menopausal hormone market. In 2001, close to 50 million Premarin prescriptions were dispensed in the United States.

Makers of Premarin and other products attempt to maximize the benefits of menopausal hormone treatment and minimize the risks and side effects. Estrogen used alone is referred to as estrogen therapy, or ET. When taken in combination with a progestin the treatment has been characterized more broadly as hormone therapy, or HT. The combination is the method of choice for women who still have their uterus intact because estrogen treatment alone can increase the risk of uterine cancer. Month after month of unopposed estrogen (without progesterone) causes excessive growth of the uterine lining, a condition known as endometrial hyperplasia, described in chapter 2. With the incessant cell divisions caused by estrogen stimulation, there is the risk of progressing from hyperplasia to adenomatous hyperplasia, a precursor to endometrial cancer. Progesteronelike hormones (progestins) protect the cells from estrogen-caused hyperstimulation. Consequently, adding progesterone or a progestin to the treatment counterbalances the growth-stimulating effect of estrogen. Combi-Patch, FemHT, Ortho-Prefest, Activella, and Prempro are some of the products now available; others are under investigation. When the estrogen and progestin are used in combination, the endometrium, instead of growing out of control, eventually shrinks and atrophies. Not only does this thwart the cancer potential of unopposed estrogen, but it also prevents endometrial bleeding. Women who want to maintain menstrual-like periods can use a progestin cyclically, taking it along with estrogen in the last 12 days of a cycle. This builds up the endometrium to some extent so when the estrogen and progestin are discontinued, a withdrawal flow follows, mimicking a menstrual period. One Premarin-containing product is packaged specifically for this purpose (PremPhase). Although this regimen results in a bleeding pattern that resembles normal menstruation, the flow occurs solely as a result of hormone treatment and is not the normal ovulation/menstruation cycle. Pseudo-periods of this type do not mean that postmenopausal women have to be concerned about the possibility of an unintended pregnancy.

There is a growing interest among women and reproductive health care providers in adding a small amount of testosterone to HT for the purpose of maintaining sexual interest and libido. The ovary usually synthesizes testosterone, but this production, like the other hormonal products of the ovary, usually decreases with menopause. A combination estrogen/testosterone pill is available. Because testosterone and most of its analogues are barely active when taken orally, the system of delivery is an important issue if a woman opts for adding testosterone or another androgen. It can be prescribed as a cream for transdermal absorption.

Different delivery systems have been developed for the administration of estrogens or progestins. Oral preparations are by far the most common mode of delivery. One popular progestin, DepoProvera, is available for use as a long-term injectable. One injection can last as long as three months. Patches, creams, and gels have been developed to deliver either estrogen or the progestin through the skin, and estrogen/progestin combinations can also be administered transdermally (Combi-Patch). These are applied at intervals of a few days or a week and used continuously. Patches containing estrogen alone are available for women who have had a hysterectomy (Climera, Estraderm, Vivelle.) Other approaches to estrogen treatment include the use of a ring placed in the vagina (Estring) from which the hormones are absorbed, or vaginal creams (Estrace, Premarin, Ortho Dienestrol) and tablets (Vagifem). The progestin can be administered via an intrauterine system as well (Mirena.) This system can last for three years.

Premarin is still the most widely prescribed estrogen for ET or HT, even though the publicity resulting from the release of the Women's Health Initiative (WHI) interim report caused an immediate drop in the rate of new prescriptions for the drug. There is no generic substitute that precisely duplicates the conjugates found in Premarin, but synthetic preparations of conjugated estrogens are available. Perhaps this distinctiveness has to do with the precise balance of estrogens extracted from the equine source or because of some undetermined factor that is maintained during the extraction period. The popularity of Premarin may have been self-generating because women have felt more secure using a product that has been on the market for more that 50 years for which hundreds of millions of prescriptions have been filled.

The release of the 2002 WHI study on the long-term effects of Prempro prompted an immediate interest in the other relatively new formulations that were not tested in the WHI study. In fact, these products had begun to gain a growing share of the market long before the WHI report appeared. These newer products usually contain the estrogen known as ethinyl estradiol or estradiol 17β, the hormone produced by the human ovary. They are active when taken orally but can also be used effectively by applying a skin patch. The hormone is absorbed through the skin and enters the general circulation, without passing first to the liver. There are advantages to avoiding the first pass through the liver with respect to gastrointestinal side effects and the potential of liver toxicity.

Estrogenic preparations from plant sources that can be taken in the form of pills or tablets are also available. These phytoestrogens are derived from a variety of plants, including soy products and yams. Some women find them appealing because they are "natural" and seem therefore, less potentially harmful than synthetic estrogens.

The majority of women using menopausal hormone therapy require a combination of estrogen and a progesteronelike compound because most women still have their uterus in place as they enter menopausal years and must not take the cancer risk of using unopposed estrogen. Progesterone is available for this purpose, administered by vaginal cream (Crinone.) An oral form of micronized progesterone (Prometrium) is also marketed. Most widely used, however, is a compound known as medroxyprogesterone acetate (Provera), which is frequently prescribed along with Premarin. The combination can be achieved by taking separate pills of each hormone or as a single pill called Prempro. This is the product that was tested in the WHI study that was brought to a halt prematurely. It is available in two doses of the progestin to permit some flexibility depending on a woman's response (the study tested the lower dose). The FDA has approved labeling information on its uses to include hot flashes and night sweats, vaginal dryness, and to help manage osteoporosis. The FDA believes there is adequate information to justify each of these claims.

I recall the tension-packed session of the FDA advisory committee some years ago when the sponsoring company first requested approval to market Premarin specifically labeled for hormone therapy in the menopause. The data submitted at that time justified approval of some but not all claims. Although this was a disappointment to the sponsor, our decision as FDA advisors prompted the design of studies that could provide hard data pertaining to other menopausal symptoms. This requirement does not apply to the nutritional supplements purported to be effective for the relief of menopausal symptoms because they are not regulated by the FDA.

A number of combination products include other synthetic progestins. They give women the opportunity to use progestins with long clinical histories because of their use in oral contraceptives. These products are available either for oral use (FemHRT, Activella, and Ortho-Prefest) or as a skin patch (Combi-Patch). FemHRT is a combination of ethinyl estradiol and norethindrone acetate, one of the first progestins marketed as an oral contraceptive. Activella is another oral pill that contains norethindrone acetate along with estradiol-17β. Ortho-Prefest combines one of the most modern progestins, norgestimate, with estradiol. Combi-Patch releases estradiol and norethindrone acetate through the skin into the bloodstream.

At the time of maximum usage, more than 10 million American women were taking menopausal hormone treatment every day. By 2002, an estimated two out of five women in the menopausal years were using some form of the hormone therapy. The numbers were expected to grow as the baby boomers cause an increase in the portion of population in the menopausal years.

The expected trend may not materialize, however, as anxiety concerning safety, fanned by publicity given to the WHI study released in July 2002, resulted in a decline in HT use by American women. Immediately after the report was released, new prescriptions written for HT fell more than 30% in one week. The media stories, some extreme in their hysteria, were bound to have an effect on HT, even though the risk findings were not new. Ten years earlier, an analysis of 37 original studies considered to be unbiased and of high quality concluded that HT could have a role as a breast cancer promoter but did not increase mortality from the disease. The unexpected finding concerning risk of cardiovascular events had also been foreshadowed by the findings of previous studies.

Subsequent reports from the WHI study in 2003 emphasized discouraging findings for older women regarding cognitive function, the risk of ischemic stroke, and relief from some menopausal symptoms. This prompted a further decline in menopausal hormone use.

Hormonal management of menopausal symptoms has been available and utilized for more than half a century. Given that long interval, it is understandably perplexing and frustrating to women that definitive information on its use is still not complete enough to answer all questions. Just when we think we have all of the pertinent facts on which to base a decision about whether to use ET/HT, yet another study is released that demands reevaluation of the previously accepted approach.

Women should be able to depend on their doctors to keep abreast of the latest information on safety issues and to carefully judge the merits of statistics on which the claimed benefits are based. For a woman and her doctor, the problem is to settle on a program of menopause management that takes into consideration the best information available. There should be a reevaluation of the merits of continuing treatment at regular intervals. With regard to menopausal hormone therapy, there are no shortcuts; treatment of choice must be individualized.

4 • Why should women consider hormone therapy?

For most women, the onset of menopause is easily recognized. As the name implies, menstrual periods stop. This is when women first start to wonder whether they should consider hormone therapy.

Hot flashes are the symptom that most of the time prompts women to seek guidance on menopause from a doctor or other health care provider. Hot flashes are an indication of vasomotor instability causing dilation of small capillaries thought the body. This causes a sudden flushing and reddening of the face, usually accompanied by perspiration. When hot flashes occur at night, sleep is often interrupted. Many women awaken night after night, their bed drenched in perspiration. During the day, the hot flashes occur unpredictably and can be the cause of awkward social and professional situations.

At menopause, estrogen production by the ovary falls below a critical level. Hot flashes and associated sleep disturbances are caused by this estrogen deprivation. Many scientific studies have shown conclusively that estrogen administration prevents hot flashes. These studies have compared the effectiveness of placebos and estrogen and find an enormous difference. Symptoms are controlled in almost all estrogen users. For women who choose not to use estrogens or any other therapy, hot flashes usually last from one to two years before abating spontaneously, but about 25% find that the condition persists for five years or longer.

The unquestionable effect of estrogen on vasomotor phenomena such as hot flashes, sleep deprivation, and alertness has led to the claim that hormone therapy (HT) can "improve the quality of life." Women who have experienced this benefit would certainly endorse this claim. To jump from this claim to the idea that estrogen forever will invariably keep women more youthful, active, or vibrant is an overstatement. A beneficial therapy for some women cannot become a panacea for all women. No one who thinks seriously about hormone therapy believes this, but press reports continue to surface that question the merit of HT because it is not a fountain of youth. Usually these news items are based on articles in the medical literature that need more careful and critical analysis than a science reporter can provide, struggling to meet a deadline for tomorrow's paper or the evening news report on television.

An example of these types of media reports involves a study done by a respected group of doctors at Stanford University School of Medicine and published in the *Journal of the American Medical Association*. The study reported on findings in nearly 3000 postmenopausal women of average age 67 with documented heart or coronary artery disease. Half received HT and the other half received placebo pills for three years. The main purpose of the study was to determine if estrogen use reduced the chances of having another adverse heart-related event. The investigators concluded that the therapy had "mixed effects on quality of life among older women." Women who had menopausal symptoms before the study benefited, while those who did not have menopausal symptoms did not benefit. In other words, if a woman doesn't have any symptoms to begin with, HT can't make her feel even better. Hormone therapy cannot make normal women more normal. The press reports, however, took a different tack. *The New York Times* headline was, "Value of Hormone Treatment Questioned." It is understandable that many women reach for the phone at once and expect reassurance from their doctors.

Data on quality of life issues were summarized in a second publication of the Women's Health Initiative in May 2003. The editors of the *New England Journal of Medicine* decided to release the study in advance of its actual publication. It was heralded in a detailed *New York Times* article with the headline, "Hormone Therapy, already found to have risks is now said to lack benefits." However, the actual findings were that women ages 50–59 who were suffering from vasomotor symptoms experienced significant symptom improvement in the Prempro group. A smaller improvement in sleep disturbances was also found. The headline refers to the overall group of study patients whose mean age on enrollment was

63. Since most of the women were no longer experiencing flashes or sleep disturbances when they entered the study, it is not at all surprising that "improvement" was marginal at best.

Estrogen is the hormone that supports and maintains the lining of the vagina. In its absence, the vaginal epithelial lining eventually becomes thin and atrophic, making penetration during sexual intercourse increasingly difficult. In extreme cases, the vagina becomes so atrophic that it narrows to less than a centimeter in diameter, entirely eliminating the possibility of normal intercourse. In an earlier time, these changes were looked upon as an inevitable sequel of the aging process, and sexual function was rarely a subject of discussion. Given the effectiveness of estrogen treatment, there is no need to tolerate painful intercourse, referred to as "dyspareunia," and sexual function can be maintained well into old age. Doctors treating menopausal women should consider sexual function and advise a woman on any sexual issues that might arise. This is especially pertinent for menopausal women who experience physical changes that may interfere with their ability to have intercourse.

I illustrate this point when teaching medical students by describing situations when women who, after many postmenopausal years without HT, establish a relationship with a man but find that without hormone therapy intercourse would be virtually impossible. After she uses vaginal estrogen, the situation can improve and the woman is able to have successful intercourse associated with complete and satisfactory response on her part.

Another important consideration is the effect of estrogen on the urinary tract. As the vagina becomes thinner, the urethra is no longer well supported. In some cases there are changes in the relationship between the urethra and the bladder itself. The net result is increasing difficulty maintaining normal urinary tract function. This is often associated with a sense of urinary urgency and occasionally even urinary incontinence. In many cases, the beneficial effect of estrogen is prompt and dramatic.

Other long-term consequences of postmenopausal lack of estrogen are now recognized as major concerns. Principal among these is osteoporosis, a thinning of the bones that can result in collapsing vertebrae and an increased risk of fracture, mainly of the hip, in older women. Osteoporosis-related fractures frequently are an indirect cause of death in older women. Fractures at this stage of life can lead to immobility, increasing, for example, the chances of blot clots or pneumonia. The National Osteoporosis Foundation guidelines urge that all women be counseled on the risk of osteoporosis. The guidelines advise that bone mineral density tests be performed on all postmenopausal women who have suffered a fracture. The foundation further recommends bone mineral density testing for any postmenopausal woman who is older than 65 with one or more risk factors for osteoporosis. The risk factors include early menopause or a history of nonpregnancy-related amenorrhea lasting more than a year, fracture as an adult, advanced age, dementia, poor health, and frailty resulting in an increased tendency to fall.

There are additional risk factors for osteoporosis that women can modify themselves, with the aid of proper counseling and guidance. Smokers have a higher risk of osteoporosis than do nonsmokers. The disease is more common in women who have more than three alcoholic drinks per day and among those that have limited physical activity. Osteoporosis is more common in women with low body weight and among women who consistently have a low calcium intake in their diet.

Hormone therapy prevents osteoporosis and reduces the risk of fracture by maintaining bone density. In normal physiology, bone density is maintained by a balance between absorption of old bone and restructuring of new bone. With aging and depletion of the body's estrogen supply, this balance tilts toward a greater degree of absorption, leaving the bone structure less dense and weaker. Estrogen therapy counteracts this by its antiabsorptive action on the bone. In the absence of osteoporosis, there is significant reduction in fracture risk. Therefore, the earlier treatment is started, the greater the protection. Furthermore, it is never too late to initiate HT to prevent future fractures. In a recent study of continuous, low-dose HT in elderly women, dramatic changes in mineral density were observed in the spine. The difference was marked when compared with the use of placebo. Both groups were treated with calcium and vitamin D. In this study, which appeared in the *Annals of Internal Medicine*, total body bone mineral density also displayed a significant increase.

In addition to hormone therapy and efforts to modify risk factors such as cigarette smoking and excessive alcohol consumption, calcium intake is important. A 1200 mg per day intake of calcium is recommended, along with 400–800 IU vitamin D per day, especially for high risk women. Calcium-rich foods, such as milk, cheese, and yogurt, can supply a good part of required calcium, but calcium supplement in the various forms available can also be useful. Toffee-like preparations rich in calcium, though costly, are popular products. Regular weight-bearing exercise is an important component of osteoporosis prevention as well.

Although HT has been proven to maintain bone mineral density and reduce the risk of fractures, there are other medications that can maintain bone mineral density with aging. These alternatives should be considered by women before deciding to use HT for the specific purpose of preventing osteoporosis. Furthermore, the importance of lifestyle pattern and diet should not be overlooked. Exercise, cessation of smoking, limiting alcohol consumption, and a calcium-rich diet are all factors within a woman's personal control that can be effective in conserving bone density with aging.

5 • Risk–benefit ratio: Making the choice

One of my patients commented as we discussed continuing her hormone therapy that whenever there are press stories about hazards of menopause treatments, cancer or otherwise, they usually related to the very medicines I was prescribing for her. I reminded her that medical articles conveying good news are rarely considered newsworthy, so she is not going to read about them in the morning paper and that nonprescription therapies unregulated by the FDA are not subjected to rigorous trial or testing, so there are rarely findings, good or bad, to write news stories about. Under these ground rules, it is a self-fulfilling prophecy that if there is a story about HT in the lay press, it is going to be scary.

There has been no shortage of attention given to the risks and benefits of HT. Here is a list of the studies funded by the National Institutes of Health and others in the recent years. Their titles describe the long list of subjects that have been studied.

HERS (Heart and Estrogen/Progestin Replacement Study)
HERS II (Heart and Estrogen/Progestin Replacement Study)
WEST (Women's Estrogen for Stroke Trial)
WHI (Women's Health Initiative)
Nurses' Health Study
HOPE (Women's Health, Osteoporosis, Progestin, Estrogen trial)
ERA (Estrogen Replacement and Atherosclerosis trial)

EPAT (Estrogen in the Prevention of Atherosclerosis Trial)
MORE (Multiple Outcomes of Raloxifene Evaluation)
PEPI (Postmenopausal Estrogen/Progestin Interventions study)
SWAN (Study of Women's Health Across the Nation)

In addition, there have been studies carried out in Europe and elsewhere.

For every treatment in medicine, the benefits need to be considered side by side with the risks. Sometimes, this is a no-brainer, especially when you have the help of FDA experts for evaluating safety and effectiveness issues and for approving information in the package labeling. But the determination of trade-offs is not always clear-cut. It is not easy for an individual woman, and it is not easy for her health care provider. Any prescription needs to be customized to fit the needs of the individual patient; this is especially true for a medication that is used long term. A woman should be involved in the decision of what an acceptable risk is, and with guidance and counseling, decide whether the treatment being considered is justified. The decision must take into account whether alternative methods exist that have the benefits important to her but that are less risky.

In the case of hormone therapy, it is not a simple yes or no question. The issue is whether to start, what product to choose, what dose to start with, and when to stop. A woman's informed participation in the decision making is essential. She should know the benefits and risks, and she should be informed about alternative therapies. Full disclosure must include the results of the WHI study released in July 2002.

Can it be claimed that there are nonhormonal approaches proven to be as effective and less risky? After the publication of the WHI, one of the weekly news magazines did a cover story entitled "Beyond HRT" and offered advice on what women could do to replace HT. The article suggested yoga for hot flashes and crossword puzzles to keep the brain alert and active. If you get this advice from your doctor, I suggest that you get a second opinion.

There is no alternative therapy that has such a documented, clinically beneficial effect on the reproductive tract, urinary tract, bone, and the brain as does estrogen. And there are other benefits of estrogen in menopause that are less familiar except to the women who have benefited from treatment. Outcomes like preventing urinary tract infections, protecting against the loss of teeth, improving wound-healing, and reducing the risk of cataract formation have been documented in the scientific literature.

The long-term benefits have important health implications for women. HT significantly reduces the risk of colon cancer and the risks of hip and vertebral fractures.

There are alternatives in modern medicine that can help specifically to preserve bone density. The prescription medication includes a group of drugs called biphosphonates (Fosamax-alendronate and Actonel-risedronate) that prevent bone resorption. These drugs can be used alone or in combination with estrogen to maintain bone density and protect against other estrogen deprivation symptoms. There is also a "designer" estrogen that protects the bones selectively (Evista-raloxifene.) Other molecules with this specificity are in the research pipeline. However, until something new comes along, the overall beneficial effects of estrogen cannot be replicated by any substitute therapy for which there is evidence-based proof of effectiveness.

For some symptoms, the benefits of estrogen with or without progestin are immediate. Women with intense menopausal symptoms, such as debilitating hot flashes, sleeplessness, or mood changes, usually experience dramatic relief. The supportive effects of estrogen on the vagina and vulva are extremely important, particularly for women for whom continued sexual function is important. Vaginal dryness resulting in painful intercourse is one of the most frequent complaints of menopausal women and can be remedied rather quickly by topical estrogens or ET.

Some menopausal women continue to produce adequate amounts of estrogen from sources other than the ovary. The adrenal gland and fat cells normally produce a small amount of estrogens. Thus, for some, the vagina remains well supported and lubricated, hot flashes are absent, and there are no sleep disturbances years after the cessation of menstruation. In these cases, a decision not to use HT is entirely reasonable, provided there is continuous monitoring and periodic evaluation for long-term complications of estrogen deprivation. Not only should bone mineral loss be carefully watched, but the possible beneficial effects of estrogens on the brain or on preventing frequent urinary tract infections should also be taken into account. Improved cognitive function may prove to be a major benefit for the long-term use of HT, but this is not scientifically established. Studies are still in progress measuring the effect of estrogen on the onset of Alzheimer's disease. So far, the evidence suggests that it may have a role in the prevention but not treatment of the disease.

The risk factors involved in using hormone replacement include some factors about which we can be certain and others that are not that certain. We know, for example, that women with an intact uterus should not take ET (so-called unopposed estrogen); this is a certainty. If a woman with an intact uterus takes estrogen, over time she may increase her risk of endometrial cancer 10-fold or more. This means her risk of developing endometrial cancer would increase from 1 in a 1000 to 1 in 100. This is an unacceptable risk, and this is why unopposed estrogen is not prescribed for most women entering the menopause. The addition of progestin, creating HT, is extremely effective in overcoming the risk of unopposed estrogen. The excess risk created by estrogen can be virtually eliminated by concurrent use of a progestin. This risk reduction occurs whether the progestin is taken continuously or cyclically.

Breast cancer risk is what most women fear and is one of the principal issues in the decision as to whether postmenopausal hormone treatment is acceptable. Studies have shown that a substantial number of prescriptions for HT remain unfilled. This is largely a measure of the intense concern of every woman over the possibility of developing breast cancer. This concern is accentuated by the extensive press coverage received by a suggestion of causal relationship between any environmental factor and breast cancer.

Cornell University maintains a bibliography on Breast Cancer and Environmental Risk Factors. As of March 2002, the section of the database on postmenopausal hormone treatment and the risk of breast cancer contained 160 articles in scientific and medical journals published just since 1995. These include clinical trials, epidemiological studies, review articles, and commentaries. The results reported are inconsistent but the general consensus has been that, with increasing time of use, there is an increased risk with estrogen alone and adding progestin is not protective. In fact, adding progestin might increase the risk slightly. Clinicians have known this for years and have insisted that HT be accompanied by annual mammograms. Some doctors instruct their patients on HT to do self-examinations regularly and report in for semiannual office appointments along with routine annual mammography. Reports that doubt the value of mammograms and self-examination of the breast should not deter women from continuing to pursue these measures that could lead to early detection.

An increased risk of breast cancer has been one of the factors taken into account in starting HT, but the extent of the increased risk has never been clear, nor have we known how to identify women with greatest risk. We know, for example, that some women carry familial genes that put them at greater risk of breast cancer. Do these women have a greater risk if they use HT? We can't be certain (the complexity and cost of doing such a study would be prohibitive), but it is prudent for women who carry the breast cancer gene to avoid any possible added risk. Even without taking HT or identifiable cancer genes into account, a woman whose mother, sister, or daughter developed breast cancer before age 40 is in a high-risk category that may increase her risk of breast cancer at least threefold. This, too, is a category of women who should avoid any added risk factors. They should avoid smoking and obesity, for example, and they should avoid taking estrogen or estrogen plus progestin for managing menopause. For some unexplained reason, women with a college education or women who reach menopause at a late age seem to have a greater chance of developing breast cancer, but it seems absurd to recommend that women in these categories should avoid HT.

The next update of the Cornell bibliography will include many new articles prompted by the WHI study report of July 2002 published in the *Journal of the American Medical Association*. This one publication appears to have superseded the entire earlier literature on breast cancer and HT because it quantifies some risks and benefits after a randomized, prospective study. In the study, hormone therapy (Prempro) was taken continuously by women, the majority of whom were at least ten years after menopause. Nearly 70% of the women enrolled were over age 60 and the average age at start of study was 63.3 years.

For this subsection of postmenopausal women, here's what the WHI study found on breast cancer: During the first four years, there was no significant difference in breast cancer rates between women using Prempro continuously and those taking placebos, but the overall risk of breast cancer diverged slightly between the two groups. By 5.2 years of use, the absolute risk in the placebo group was 30 events annually per 10,000 women. In the HT group it was 38 per 10,000. This confirms earlier observational and epidemiological studies indicating that there is a slight increase in risk that is related to the duration of use of HT.

The added risk of a diagnosis of breast cancer in the treatment group was the calculation that triggered the decision to end the WHI trial. Over the average 5.2 years of observation, the 8 additional cases of diagnosed breast cancer per 10,000 women years of use of Prempro represented an increased relative risk of 26%. This increase almost reached statistical significance but fell slightly short of that threshold. In clinical research, when a difference between two groups is not statistically significant, it means that the difference could be by chance and that if the study were repeated, it could turn out differently. In this case, the chances are that the difference is meaningful because it confirms earlier work and the time trend during the study was consistent. The risk difference, nevertheless, was small. It was less than one tenth of 1% per year.

Among the Prempro users were many older women who had previously used HT in menopause, some for longer than 10 years. Women with a history of prior use of hormone therapy had a considerably higher incidence of breast cancer diagnosis by the time the study was stopped than women who had no history of hormone therapy use before entering the study. In addition to many years of hormone use before entering the study, prior-users in the treatment group received hormones during the study's 5.2 years. By design, the 8102 placebo users had no hormone exposure during the study. When the study ended, the 6280 women (out of the total group of 8502) who had never used postmenopausal hormones before receiving the Prempro pills handed out during the study had a statistically insignificant 6% increase in the rate of diagnosis of breast cancer, compared to the placebo group. Only when the 2222 prior-users in the Prempro group are added to the calculation does the risk hazard approach the level of statistical significance.

The widely publicized WHI finding of a 26% increase in the risk of breast cancer applies only if women who are prior users of menopausal hormone therapy are included in the calculations. It does not apply to women who are just entering menopause and have not used hormone therapy previously. For them, there is minimal chance of incurring an increased risk of breast cancer, according to the WHI study.

The study did not find a difference in breast cancer mortality rates between the HT group and the placebo group. In fact the overall death rates between the two groups did not differ. This, too, is a confirmation of earlier information. For example, in 1992, 37 publications in the scientific literature considered to be of high quality and unbiased were combined for further analysis (called a meta-analysis) and it was concluded that HT might act as a breast cancer promoter. But the analysis also concluded that the therapy did not increase deaths due to breast cancer and could have a net beneficial effect on mortality. The WHI study also found that all-cause mortality did not differ between the groups using HT or placebo pills during the 5-plus years of follow-up. This may be because the time was too short to reveal mortality rate differences but the same concern about timing raises uncertainty whether the cancers reported in the WHI study were actually started by the treatment. Five years may be too short a time to expect to see a difference in mortality rates, but it is also a very short time for newly formed cancer to reach a size that could be diagnosed. Oncologists believe this usually takes at least 10 years. Rather than discovering new tumors, the annual examinations during the course of the study may have disclosed preexisting cancers brought up to detectable size by the hormone stimulation whether they had initially been caused by earlier HT exposure or some other environmental or genetic factor. A follow-up published in June 2003 analyzed the characteristics of breast cancers observed in the WHI study and the record of mammography results. The authors concluded that estrogen plus progestin may stimulate breast cancer growth, as previously reported, and may cause a delay in breast cancer diagnosis using mammography. This is valuable information in the fight against breast cancer but it adds a new piece to the puzzle. Breast cancer mortality rates in the United States have been steadily declining in the recent decades of growing use of both HT and mammography. Advances in treatment play a vital role in saving the lives of many women with this dreadful disease, but regular screening and early diagnosis also help to reduce mortality from breast cancer.

The WHI has not reported that estrogen therapy without progestin (ET) presents a significant excess risk of breast cancer compared to the placebo group.

The U.S. FDA requires that prescription drug labeling include contraindications to the use of a product. This is the most serious of the categories of alerts about risks associated with the use of a medication. Lesser concerns are listed under the categories of warnings or precautions. Several definite contraindications are listed for HT. Among these is a known or suspected pregnancy. As medical students before the era of menstruation-suppressing contraceptives, we were taught that any woman of reproductive age with amenorrhea should be considered pregnant until proved otherwise. This includes women approaching menopause, although the likelihood of a pregnancy beyond the age of 45 is extremely low. Nevertheless, any woman who has any reason to believe that cessation of menstruation may due to an unexpected conception should test for pregnancy. The availability of home pregnancy tests makes this uncomplicated and private. The risks that worry the FDA are an undetected ectopic pregnancy that might go untreated and the possible deleterious effects of the hormones on the developing fetus.

A second absolute contraindication to HT is known or suspected breast cancer, endometrial cancer, or any tumor that may be estrogen dependent. When a reproductive system cancer is suspected, tests must be carried out to establish or rule out the diagnosis before proceeding with any use of hormones. The reason for this is that the exogenous hormones would enhance tumor growth. Some breast cancers are not estrogen-sensitive because they test negative for the presence of estrogen receptors. In these cases, there is a reasonable degree of certainty that estrogen plays no role in the initiation or stimulation of the tumor. In these cases it would not be unreasonable to use a limited low-dose course of estrogen replacement when severe symptoms of hot flashes cannot be controlled by other means.

Another contraindication to HT is undiagnosed abnormal vaginal bleeding. If there has been abnormal menstruation, especially if the bleeding is heavy, a woman should not start HT until a diagnosis has been established. This usually means that the endometrium should be sampled at least by an endometrial biopsy, and possibly by dilation and curettage (D&C) to obtain more tissue in order to be sure that there is no cancer or precancerous condition of the endometrium. Sometimes, measuring the thickness of the endometrium by using transvaginal ultrasonography can suggest the diagnosis. The possibility of cervical cancer needs to be ruled out as well, and Pap smears should be obtained routinely.

The other condition in the FDA's list of definite contraindications to HT is active thrombophlebitis or thromboembolic disorders. These are blood-clotting conditions that can be life threatening. Women who have had an episode of venous thrombophlebitis, a condition which involves the lodging of clotted blood in the deep peripheral veins, mainly the veins of the legs, should not use HT. When the acute condition is evident, it requires immediate treatment. If left untreated, venous thrombophlebitis can result in blood clots migrating to the lung (pulmonary embolism), which can be fatal. Thrombophlebitis is seen with increased frequency in patients who are sedentary. Airline passengers on long flights, for example, have to be reminded to move the legs and flex the muscles of the calves from time to time to avoid pooling of blood, thrombosis, and embolism.

There has been evidence that venous thromboembolism is increased among women receiving estrogen and progestin therapy. This has been verified by the WHI study. In the WHI study, the rate of thromboembolism (venous thrombosis and pulmonary embolism) increased from 16 per 10,000 years of use to 34 per 10,000 years. This means that a woman's risk is doubled. In terms of absolute risk, it means that if a thousand untreated women are observed for 10 years, 16 will have a blot clot condition during the decade. A thousand women using HT for 10 years would result in 34 cases of thrombosis.

Whether the same results could be expected with other products or other doses of the estrogen progestin combination studied in the WHI study (Prempro at the 0.625/2.5 mg dose) cannot be certain. There could be a different effect on clotting among the various progestins used in either oral contraceptives or HT. In 1997 the World Health Organization (WHO) published the results of a study comparing newer products that contain third-generation progestins with earlier products containing other progestins. The main finding was that birth control pills with third-generation progestins seemed to be associated with a slightly higher risk of clotting disorders. Other statisticians were quick to criticize the study for failing to point out that women using the same pills had, as a group, fewer heart attacks. The changes in the statistics on either issue were extremely modest, and no products were withdrawn from the market after the results of the study were carefully analyzed. At most, some changing in the wording of patient information in product packages resulted.

Another prospective evaluation of this issue is the Heart and Estrogen/Progesterone Replacement Study (HERS). In a preliminary finding, the incidence of an initial episode of venous thromboembolism following the use of HT was small. Unexplained venous embolism is not common in women over 50 years of age. The absolute risk, which considers the underlying rate of a condition in a population, is what is important in formulating a risk–benefit ratio. The HERS study found that for every 10,000 years of use, a risk of 2 additional cases of venous thrombosis could occur. When the HERS study was extended for an additional two years, the difference between the HT group and the placebo group was larger. In the 2002 WHI report, there was an excess risk over the placebo group of 8 cases of venous thrombosis per 10,000 women-years of use.

Other studies show an association between thrombophlebitis or pulmonary embolism with the use of estrogen alone. Premenopausal women who have medical reasons for removal of their ovaries understandably wish to avoid surgically induced menopause so they may be eager to start estrogen treatment. The immediate post-operative period when the woman is still in bed is not the time to do this.

Over the years, observational studies have reported a decreased risk of mortality from coronary heart disease in HT users. This decrease is reported variously between 35% and 50%, but because these are mainly observational studies, and not long-term, prospective, and randomized with adequate control groups, their results are not definitive. Nevertheless, the amount of data has been impressive. In 1992 a meta-analysis, which combines for reanalysis the results of many smaller studies, concluded that estrogen reduces risks for coronary heart disease about 35%.

The Nurse's Health Study, centered at Harvard's Brigham and Women's Hospital, has been in progress since 1976 collecting health reports from women on an ongoing basis. It is the largest database ever assembled to analyze the etiology of major diseases. A 1996 report on more than 400,000 woman years of follow-up concluded that women on HT had a 40–60% reduction in cardiovascular events. Since heart disease is the leading cause of death in postmenopausal women, the importance of documenting with certainty the heart benefits of HT was one of the major reasons for starting the WHI study in 1993.

Although the WHI study was designed to be a random assignment double blind study, considered to be the gold standard of clinical trials, this does not mean that it was representative of the general population that might use hormone therapy. As explained in the commentary, women with extreme symptoms of menopause (hot flashes, night sweats, vaginal irritation, incontinence, or sleeplessness) were excluded on an ethical basis since it would be difficult for them clinically if they were randomly assigned to the placebo group and did not receive any treatment for their complaints. However, these are precisely the women for whom most prescriptions for HT are written. Eighty-five percent of prescriptions for Prempro and similar products are for less-than-five-year users who are taking HT for quality of life symptoms. This exclusion criterion eliminated from the study mainly women just entering menopause so that the average age of the WHI study group, at 63.2 years, was older than newly menopausal women in general. Consequently, the preexistence of other diseases of aging, including early stages of atherosclerosis, was hard to exclude. About one-third of the women in the study were being treated for hypertension and 69% were overweight. Preexisting heart disease or diabetes was reported by 13% of the women.

There is a theoretical basis for a cardio-protective effect of HT. In long-term studies in women treated with a variety of hormone replacement treatments, including estrogen and a progestin in various combinations, a significant increase has been observed in the level of high-density lipoprotein (HDL), the good cholesterol, with a significantly decreased level of the bad cholesterol, low-density lipoprotein (LDL). Both ET and HT have this beneficial effect, but estrogen without progestin causes an even greater increase in HDL. Everything we know about cholesterol and clogging of blood vessels teaches us that this is bound to be a heart-friendly property of ET or HT. There have been randomized placebo-controlled studies of drugs that reduce cholesterol showing that the risk of heart disease is reduced.

Estrogen not only slows development of atherosclerosis (clogging of arteries due to plaque formation), but it can also impede arteriosclerosis (hardening of the arteries). A Mayo Clinic study found that women who take estrogen decrease their risk of the progressive narrowing and hardening of the arteries. The calcium content of the coronary arteries in women using ET was 90% lower than in postmenopausal women not taking ET, and cholesterol plaque formation was not increased compared to premenopausal women. These vascular changes would result in decreased lipid accumulation in the coronary arteries and decreased loss of vascular flexibility caused by calcium deposition.

In spite of these desirable cardiovascular actions of estrogen, observations on about 2400 women in the Heart and Estrogen/progestin Replacement Study (HERS) did not find a beneficial effect of estrogen for women who had already had a primary coronary heart disease (CHD) event. In the study, women were randomized to a group treated with estrogen/progestin and one treated with a placebo. There was an increased relative hazard in the HT treated group after one year, but the risk decreased in time thereafter. By years four and five, HT users had a substantially reduced risk of a primary heart disease event (angina, shortness of breath) or of a nonfatal myocardial infarction (heart attack).

The larger WHI Study, however, found no heart-protective effect among women on HT up to 5.2 years, when the estrogen and progestin portion of the study was stopped. The overall rate of women experiencing CHD events was low, but there were 7 excess cases per 10,000 as compared with nontreated controls. The desirable changes in the lipid profile were, however, observed in the treated group. This observation remains an enigma. There is a plausible theory based mainly on animal studies but confirmed by observations in people. Tom Clarkson is a pathologist who studies the interior lining of the coronary arteries. This is the microscopic portion that thickens when there is cholesterol plaque deposition, restricting blood flow and leading to a possible heart attack. Clarkson has found that as women age the structure of plaques in the coronary arteries is altered in a manner that increases the likelihood of a clot breaking loose and leading to a heart attack. Consequently the fact that nearly 70% of the WHI population was in the older age group may have been a factor in the rate of cardiovascular adverse events in spite of the favorable changes in blood lipid patterns.

The information from the important Nurse's Health Study showing a heart-benefit effect of HT after the first year of use might be explained on the basis of age or on nonrandomness in the nature of the women reporting. Nurses tended to be more health-conscious and more educated than the population at large, so the explanation may be not that HT caused better health, but that healthy women used HT. Does this mean that results from the large, random-assignment placebo control WHI study may not pertain to the younger menopausal woman who has regular doctor's appointments, follows advice on preventive health care, eats a balanced diet, and practices other good health measures? It's a debatable question.

If you think all of this is confusing, you are not alone. In an analysis published in the cardiology journal, *Circulation*, Michael Mendelsohn and Richard Karas of Tufts University Medical School tried to bring clarity to this complicated situation. Regarding the HERS study data mentioned above, they pointed out that it teaches only that women with known cardiovascular disease who are 20 years past menopause ought not to have HT added to their medications. They emphasize the clear take-home message: For postmenopausal women, HT is not the treatment of choice to lower cholesterol levels or to protect the heart of women already suffering from cardiovascular disease. There is no substitute for good cardiovascular care. For all women, estrogen or estrogen and progestin should not be used for the prevention of cardiovascular disease.

Breast and endometrial cancers are not the only cancer-related matters related to HT. The risk of cancer is always the first concern of women considering HT, and it is wise for each woman to consider her particular risk factors. There are both encouraging and cautionary considerations about cancer to take into account. Epidemiological studies demonstrate a significant preventive effect of HT on colorectal cancer. Three independent studies found that relative risk of developing either colon or rectal cancer was significantly decreased in women using HT. Colorectal cancer (which includes cancers of both the colon and rectum) is the third leading cause of cancer-related deaths in the United States. Only lung and breast cancer claim more lives. All available evidence points to a reduction in the incidence and mortality from colorectal cancer by the use of HT. In the 2002 WHI study, hormone therapy reduced colorectal cancer by 6 cases per 10,000. This 40% reductions compared to placebo users nearly balanced out the higher incidence of breast cancer, which was increased by 8 cases per 10,000.

The relationship between HT/ET and ovarian cancer is a subject of continuing research. One large epidemiologic study carried out by the U.S. National Cancer Institute suggests a relationship between past estrogen use and ovarian cancer. Women using estrogen only, especially those who used it for more than 10 years, were at significantly increased risk. When estrogen was used in combination with a progestin, however, the relative risk was substantially less. In another study, no increased risk was observed in women who had used a progestin with the estrogen for at least 15 days each month over many years. The WHI found no difference in the diagnosis of ovarian, endometrial, or other cancers between HT users and placebo users.

The decision to use hormones to manage postmenopausal symptoms is very individual. There are significant advantages to HT/ET in terms of comfort of living and bodily functions, and there are long-term health benefits such as osteoporosis prevention. As more information is accumulated, there may be the bonus of a positive effect on brain function, including the delay in the onset of Alzheimer's disease.

The risks, particularly the increased chance of breast cancer and of blood clots, are not insignificant and must certainly be carefully considered before starting HT and should influence the length of time that the treatment is continued. The best plan for women on HT is to review the situation with their physician each year before deciding to continue.

6 • Can HT protect brain function and prevent Alzheimer's disease?

The commonly held belief that there is decreased cognitive function (mental acuity) with age is justified, but there is great individual variation. Some mental processes do slow down with age, but many do not. Studies from several countries including the United States have reached this conclusion. Research into aging has been greatly advanced by the Study of Aging in America program sponsored for more than a decade by Chicago's MacArthur Foundation. As part of this research, millions of dollars were provided to scientists and doctors around the country to support studies on aging within their particular areas of expertise. John Rowe and Robert Kahn present the results of the Aging in America Study in their book, *Successful Aging*.

Fears of mental decline, loss of memory, and especially of Alzheimer's disease are widespread among older people. According to the Aging in America study, about 10% of people over the age of 65 may have Alzheimer's disease, and the proportion increases with age. Among the oldest, people from 85 to 100 years of age or more, as many as 50% may have some degree of Alzheimer's. These are probably reliable statistics; specialists believe that cognitive tests and medical examinations now available enable them to make a diagnosis with 90% confidence.

One major component of the Aging in America Study examined how the mental function of a large group of people changed over a period of

28 years. The study measured several mental functions including the ability to use words and numbers accurately, to interpret spatial relationships among different shapes, and to interpret facts. The study found that older people definitely lose some mental ability, but even in the oldest group, half of the people showed no mental decline whatsoever. What factors enable some people to retain their mental ability with age? The idea that this retention of mental function is entirely genetic is an oversimplification. The Aging in America Study emphasizes the importance of lifestyle decisions, but physiological and hormonal factors cannot be overlooked.

Because Alzheimer's disease often surfaces initially in postmenopausal women, it has long been suspected that there may be a link between estrogen deprivation and the disease. This concept is supported by many reports in scientific journals that ET or HT forestalls the expected decline in cognitive function. But these are mainly observational studies with small numbers of cases. In one pilot study mentioned in the Rowe and Kahn book, five out of six women who had mild Alzheimer's disease improved in verbal memory and attention after using an estrogen patch for two months. Another small study done at the University of Southern California measured the cognitive performance of 36 women with clinically diagnosed Alzheimer's disease, 9 of whom were receiving estrogen therapy. To make the comparison meaningful, the treated and untreated groups were matched as carefully as possible by age, education, and duration of dementia. Results showed that women receiving estrogen therapy performed significantly better than other women on some tasks. The largest group difference was in a word memory task. The authors of this clinical report conclude that their findings support the hypothesis that estrogen therapy for women with Alzheimer's disease is associated with better cognitive skills. In another study involving more than 180 postmenopausal women in the estrogen-treated group, learning and verbal memory were markedly improved compared to the nontreated controls.

A larger study at Columbia University in New York City followed more than 1000 elderly women initially free of Alzheimer's over a range of 5 years. The relative risk of developing the disease was reduced, and the average age of onset of Alzheimer's was significantly higher in women who used estrogen replacement after the onset of menopause. The Columbia doctors concluded that estrogen use in postmenopausal women may delay the onset and decrease the risk of Alzheimer's disease.

Observational studies of this type, encouraging though they may be, cannot be considered definitive because there may be other, unidentified factors. It would be helpful if we had information from a long-term, random-assignment, placebo-controlled study that evaluated brain functions and the onset of Alzheimer's disease in women. There is one huge study in progress observing the postmenopausal experience of nearly 100,000 women with or without the use of HT, but it will not report conclusive results until 2005. This is an observational study and is part of the U.S. National Institutes of Health's Women's Health Initiative (WHI) established in 1991 and planned to continue for 15 years.

An interim report from the clinical trial of the WHI concluded that hormone use (Prempro) increases the risk of dementia in women 65 years or older. The increased risk observed resulted in 23 additional cases of dementia per 10,000 women per year. The cognitive functions measured may have no relation to Alzheimer's disease or other forms of dementia, according to the authors of the report. This may explain why the findings are the direct opposite of a study involving more than 5000 women that took place between 1995 and 2000. The authors of this study (the Cache County study) concluded that HT may protect against Alzheimer's disease. They speculate that the greatest beneficial effect may occur if HT is initiated at menopause when the sudden drop in the woman's estrogen production may have a damaging effect on the nerve cells of the brain.

We should not ignore the quality and importance of smaller observational studies of women who use ET. We can also glean useful information from laboratory and animal studies. Direct measurements of the clinical effects of estrogen on brain function are important to consider, and neurologists now have the means to do this. Alzheimer's disease is associated with deposition plaques of beta amyloid, a protein, in the brain cells. These plaques interfere with the ability of the brain cells to communicate with each other. Brain function is impaired as a result. The plaques can be visualized with an MRI brain scan so that the progression of the disease can be followed by serial comparison of scans over time.

Animal models have been developed to explore the relationship between plaque deposition and estrogen. In the guinea pig, for example, plaque deposition is increased after removal of the ovaries, and this increase can be prevented by concomitant estrogen administration. Animal studies, however, cannot be automatically carried over to humans so it is important to evaluate observations made by neuroscientists studying patients.

The effect of estrogen on the brain in women with cerebral vascular disease has been evaluated using a variety of techniques. One approach measures blood flow through the brain. A study of postmenopausal women with cerebral vascular disease found that estrogen use is associated with a trend toward increased cerebral blood flow and concluded that ET enhances cognition significantly. When brain scans, using positron emission tomography (PET), were used to study brain physiology, a decreased blood flow to a portion of the brain, the hippocampus, was found to be characteristic of Alzheimer's disease. Over a two-year interval, HT users exhibited higher hippocampus blood flow, as measured by the PET scans, as well as higher scores for memory tests. These neurophysiological studies teach us a great deal about estrogen and brain function.

Another line of sophisticated research finds that estrogen protects the brain against sudden oxygen deprivation. This is extremely important because the neuronal cells of the brain are committed to self-destruct when there is a drop in the oxygen supply. Once this process is triggered, the cells are programmed to take it to completion. This form of cell suicide "apoptosis" that begins when the oxygen supply is abruptly cut off can be forestalled by the protective effect of circulating estrogen.

The influence of estrogen on brain functions other than cognition has also been studied. This information provides indirect evidence for the hypothesis that estrogen can have a supportive role in the cognitive functions. The adrenal glands produce cortisol in increased amounts in response to stress. This is part of the body's fight-or-flight reaction to imminent danger. In an imaginative study, cortisol released from the adrenals was measured in response to stress in estrogen-treated women and in randomly selected controls. The stress in this case was exposure to a repetitive, annoying background noise. The brain performance test was a standard arithmetical problem. The estrogen-treated group exhibited no change in cortisol production, whereas in the nontreated controls there was a significant increase in cortisol. Test performance results of the nontreated controls were lower compared to the ET group. The interpretation is that ET improves the ability to accommodate stress. In a similar study, postmenopausal women experiencing marked vasomotor symptoms were evaluated for their ability to respond to stress before and after eight weeks of estrogen therapy. In this case, the hot flashes and other vasomotor symptoms were the stress. After estrogen therapy, cortisol release was significantly reduced, indicating an improved capacity to manage stress. This study confirmed that estrogen has a positive affect on the brain's ability to handle stress and on cognitive function in general.

There are literally hundreds of small observational studies, clinical laboratory studies, or animal studies that point to the association between estrogen use and improved brain function, including cognition. Estrogen has been shown to have an effect on neurotransmitters in the brain that influence mood. This helps explain why estrogen deprivation is sometimes associated with the onset of severe depression. Postpartum depression, which can have catastrophic results for a new mother and her family, occurs shortly after delivery when estrogen levels are distinctly depressed. The mood changes of premenstrual syndrome are also synchronized with the low estrogen phase of a woman's hormonal cycle.

The estrogen deprivation feature of menopause might be expected to have the same association with depression and mood changes, but the scientific evidence on this topic is mixed. Although epidemiological studies do not show an association between menopause and a higher incidence of major depression, estrogen therapy can provide relief for menopausal women already suffering from major depression. In one study improvement occurred in 68% of depressed women who were treated for 12 weeks with transdermal estrogen as compared with improvement in 20% of women in the placebo group. Mood improvement has been studied as well. In one placebo-controlled, prospective study, women receiving estrogen or estrogen plus androgen displayed significantly better mood scores than did the placebo controls. In another randomized controlled trial, asymptomatic postmenopausal women exhibited lower depression scores and improved mood with estrogen therapy. Nevertheless, with our present state of knowledge, women would certainly want to seek medical advice for conventional treatments that are available for depression.

Does estrogen slow the onset of Alzheimer's disease and protect brain function in menopausal women? Although there is a plethora of scientific studies on the subject of estrogens and the brain, extrapolating from them to a definitive answer is not justified at this point. Some have had encouraging results, and others have failed to confirm the association. Some studies have concluded that HT/ET does not slow the progression of the disease once diagnosed. One study even suggests that Hawaiin women of Japanese origin who have a diet high in soybean curd, which is rich in phytoestrogens, are more likely to develop Alzheimer's than women with a lower intake of bean curd.

Ultimately, it may take a large, long-term, placebo-controlled, random assignment, double-blind epidemiological study to answer the question to everyone's satisfaction, and even then, the benefits would have to be weighed against the possible risks.

The WHI study might have provided such information, but brain function was not one of the bodily responses it was initially designed to evaluate. When the randomized controlled clinical trial was started in 1993, earlier observational evidence of a beneficial effect of estrogen on brain function existed and might have been an incentive to consider testing for brain function effects in addition to the other benefits and risks the massive study is attempting to measure. This subject was not introduced into the study until three years after it started. Now that the estrogen-plus-progestin arm of the study has been terminated, the prospective data are shorter in duration of use and limited to women 65–70 years old. So, even after reports from the WHI study, the question of estrogen and brain function remains unresolved. It would take at least 10 years and millions of dollars to get an optimal answer; perhaps we never will. The estrogen-alone arm of the WHI random assignment clinical trial is continuing, and we may get some useful information on the subject from large data banks collected by state health departments or federal agencies that track women's health issues. Meanwhile, women and physicians will have to use their best judgment based on observational studies and other scientific information available.

In spite of the intriguing prospect of a positive effect, in the absence of long-term prospective information from well-designed studies, women would be ill-advised to use HT for the primary purpose of preventing Alzheimer's disease or for treating a mood disorder or depression. Beneficial effects on brain function, however, may prove to be a bonus benefit for women who have elected to start and continue hormone replacement at the onset of menopause.

7 • Does the approach of menopause mean the end of fertility?

There is an age-related decrease in fertility. As the biological clock ticks toward the menopausal years, women have a lower and lower chance of becoming pregnant, regardless of whether this probability is calculated on the basis of an annual or monthly chance of establishing a pregnancy by age or on the basis of chances of conception with a single act of sexual intercourse. Fertility potential declines rapidly after the age of 35 and even more dramatically after 40 (table 7.1).

At the start of perimenopause, the irregularity of ovulation begins to lower fertility: the fewer the eggs, the fewer the opportunities to establish a pregnancy. However, even perimenopausal women who continue to have regular menstrual periods find that their fertility is substantially reduced. For a long time scientists, unable to come up with a provable theory to explain this, shrugged it off as the "aging egg" phenomenon, with no further elucidation of why it happens. Now, research is delving into more rational and detailed explanations.

As new assisted reproduction techniques for infertility management have emerged, it has become clear that subfertility in ovulatory women in the late reproductive years is the direct result of biochemical and structural changes in the eggs that are being released. The eggs of older women begin to lose their fertilization potential, and, even when they

Table 7.1. Chance of a Pregnancy with Each Monthly Attempt During a Normal Cycle or an Assisted Cycle

Age of woman (years)	Pregnancy success (%)
15	22
20	24
25	25
30	17
35	8
40	3
45	<1

can be penetrated by a sperm, the resulting embryos are associated with a higher incidence of abnormal development and subsequent pregnancy loss. Miscarriages and spontaneous abortions rates increase with the age of the mother. The reason for the gradual aging of the egg is not understood, but there are various theories that scientists are testing. The aging of eggs may be the result of changes in the egg membrane, which is the entry point of sperm during fertilization, or the result of changes in the egg's cytoplasm. Since aging affects not only the egg's ability to become fertilized, but also the ultimate success of a pregnancy, scientists believe that aging changes occur within the egg itself, not simply in its membrane.

Society's concern about fertility in perimenopausal women has been heightened as increasing numbers of women have elected to postpone childbearing until the late reproductive years. The main concern about late fertility used to be that a late-in-life pregnancy would unexpectedly occur just as the kids were ready to go off to college. Now, the problem confronting many women is that postponing childbearing carries with it a risk of future infertility. Women make their own decisions on lifestyles and priorities based on their goals and personal aspirations. Some choose careers that require them to postpone having children.

I have many patients in my practice who have elected to undergo conservative procedures that can allow them to retain their fertility even though childrearing is not a part of their immediate life plans. Examples of such situations are women who at a young age develop uterine myomas or fibroids that cannot be treated medically and require surgery. Since these women, many in their late 20s or early 30s, wish to retain their fertility potential, they are successfully treated by myomectomy, the removal of the myomas with conservation of the uterus and ovaries. Usually reproductive potential can be preserved and maintained. In many of these cases, the woman's life situation is such that a pregnancy soon after the surgery is not a reasonable option. She may still be pursuing an active career or continuing graduate study, or she may have not found the right partner. Some women may eventually consider single parenthood and the use of donor insemination.

The age at which ovulation ceases varies. As menopause approaches, ovulation is no longer occurring at all or only sporadically, few eggs remain, and the chance of pregnancy becomes extremely low. This is particularly difficult for women who have premature menopause and cease to ovulate early in their reproductive life. Premature ovarian failure is an infrequent occurrence that affects about 1 woman in 300. In some cases, there is a genetic cause for the condition, but in the majority of cases it remains unexplained. In this case, in vitro fertilization (IVF) using donor eggs can give the woman a chance to become pregnant. A postmenopausal woman whose uterus is still present can sustain a pregnancy and proceed through labor and delivery because the uterus retains its functional capacity long after menopause. Because estrogen is markedly diminished in menopause, the endometrium, the uterine lining, becomes thin and inactive. Even after many years, the endometrium can be "reawakened" with the use of estrogen and progesterone, and menstrual periods can be induced almost indefinitely. The endometrium that is stimulated with estrogen and progesterone is capable of supporting the embryo and fetus throughout pregnancy. An egg from a donor can be fertilized in vitro using either a husband's or a donor's sperm, and three to four days later the resulting embryo is transferred to the uterus. Meanwhile the prospective mother has received hormone treatments that simulate a natural ovulatory cycle (estrogen first, then progesterone) so that her uterus is prepared to accept the embryo. The overall success rate following this treatment is even higher than with standard IVF procedures probably because the eggs that are used are obtained from young volunteers and are substantially more fertilizable than those that can be recovered from women in the late reproductive years.

The use of donor eggs has enabled women whose ovaries are no longer functional or even present to have a baby. This approach has been referred to as "semiadoption" because the couple has "adopted" the egg. When use of this procedure began, there was considerable controversy. There are still those who, usually for religious reasons, find the use of a donor egg, or, for that, matter donor sperm, to be unacceptable. Others, however, have no philosophical problem with the use of donor gametes (eggs and sperm) and are grateful for the opportunity to establish a pregnancy. The Hebrew University's Hadassah Medical School's successful program in assisted reproduction is greatly appreciated by Israeli couples with impaired fertility. It was there that Joseph Schenker and his team carried out the first successful IVF procedure using a donor egg, having considered the ethical issues extensively before proceeding.

There are important differences between the use of donor eggs and the use of donor sperm. Sperm collection is a simple matter with no risk to the donor. Collection of eggs from the donor requires a series of technical procedures that are not without risk. For the recovery of eggs, the donor must be treated with hormones, first to suppress her ovulation, then to stimulate the development of ovarian follicles that contain the eggs, using follicle stimulating hormone. Ovulation is then triggered with yet another hormone, luteinizing hormone or human chorionic gonadotropin. The eggs are recovered from the donor by passing a needle through the vagina into each follicle and aspirating the follicles one by one. Ovarian stimulation is relatively safe, but nevertheless it is associated with occasional complications that are serious. The egg recovery also is reasonably safe, but, in rare cases, can be complicated by infection, which has the potential of affecting future reproductive capacity. There are certainly emotional considerations surrounding the donation of eggs. Consider, for example, the woman who decides to donate eggs while a college student, who later in life experiences infertility herself. These issues notwithstanding, donor egg programs are now well established. The best of these include a requirement for extensive pretreatment counseling and informed consent.

Another issue that may never be resolved satisfactorily concerns the level of financial compensation received by an egg donor. Ethics committees have taken the position that compensation should be solely for time and effort required for the procedures and counseling. Selling of human tissue and organs, including sperm, eggs or embryos, has been deemed unethical. In fact, it is illegal in most countries. There is a fine line between reasonable compensation and coercion through financial incentive, but it is a difficult line to tread. College newspapers and other publications are replete with ads recruiting egg donors with offers of large amounts of money for "the right" donor, with qualifications outlined such as high SAT scores, attractive appearance, and the like. It doesn't take a Ph.D. in bioethics to reject this misuse of assisted reproduction.

Egg donation, initially used only to treat patients with absent ovaries or premature menopause, has been applied for other purposes. From at least three countries, pregnancies have been reported in women in their 60s. Those who take the position that this matter should be one of personal choice and outsiders have no right to interfere, claim a double standard is being applied since no one raises ethical or cultural objections to pregnancies in couples whose male partner is in his 60s. The name of some famous entertainer invariably comes up as an example in these arguments.

From a medical point of view, the principal ethical issue is that of informed consent. How can we determine a risk level and properly advise a 60-year-old woman who wishes to establish a pregnancy with donor eggs? So few cases have been reported that it is impossible to know how risky this procedure is. As is the case in so many other clinical situations, common sense should apply. Certainly there is always some risk of health complications in a pregnancy, but for women in their 50s and 60s, when the incidence of heart disease and thrombosis rises sharply, it is obvious that these risks would be increased. Consider, for example, the 60-year-old woman who elects to proceed with a pregnancy and during the course of that pregnancy suffers a stroke or a fatal embolus or a convulsion resulting from uncontrolled hypertension.

The level of uncertainty is even greater for the developing fetus. There is virtually no information on the effect of maternal age on the function of the placenta as it develops. The overriding question is whether the placenta is impaired as a result of maternal aging. We do know that there is an increased incidence of fetal growth retardation in women over 40. It stands to reason that with a woman's increasing age there is an increased incidence of atherosclerosis, which would compromise circulation to the uterus, and a greater incidence of such conditions as adult-onset diabetes. Therefore, it is not unreasonable to assume that placental blood circulation, essential for the delivery of oxygen and nutrients to the fetus, might in some cases be impaired when women become pregnant in their 50s and 60s. The production of pregnancies in postmenopausal women by assisted reproduction techniques is an experiment that is fraught with uncertainty. A woman should consider overall risks and benefits for herself, and fetal well-being is a separate issue that must also be taken into account.

In an effort to improve the quality of eggs recovered from older women, methods are being explored to treat the egg itself. One such approach involves inserting cytoplasm, the cellular component that surrounds the egg nucleus, from a young donor egg into an aging one. The egg nucleus contains the chromosomes, and initially it was thought that injection of young cytoplasm would not transmit heritable material. Recently, however, it has been shown that some DNA from the donor is, in fact, transferred into the egg of the recipient when cytoplasmic transfer is done. These experiments, although resulting in healthy offspring, are recent, and it is impossible at this point to guarantee that the child will not exhibit abnormalities later in life. These considerations would make the use of donor eggs a more reasonable and safer option than cytoplasmic transfer.

In the natural course of events, a woman's fertility declines with advancing years, pregnancy is extremely unlikely during perimenopause, and fertility is lost along with ovarian function in menopause. As women wish to delay child bearing, the advances of assisted reproduction technology adds a postscript to the idea that fertility ends according to a preset biological clock. In discussing fertility potential with patients who have had a reproductive problem and who are older than 35, I advise that sooner is better than later. The comment I have heard so often is, "that is all very well, but pregnancy with whom?"

8 • Herbal products for menopause

Doctors are usually unwilling to make recommendations that are not based on evidence. Our professional decisions are guided by the information and experience of modern medicine, arguably the best and most sophisticated the world has ever known. Sometimes, this elicits the criticism that we medicalize conditions that are a normal part of life. Disapproval is leveled particularly at medical management of the menopause, an event which predictably occurs in the lives of all women who survive into their 50s and beyond. The complaint is that many health care providers are likely to recommend hormone treatment without considering other options, while failing to provide common-sense guidance on healthy living and preventive measures that have stood the test of time.

Many women are skeptical about hormones and react by seeking alternative approaches to manage the symptoms of the menopause. These include relaxation techniques, chiropractic massage, herbal medicines, and megavitamins. In a survey of menopausal women, as many as four out of five indicated that they had used nonprescription remedies to manage both the short-term and long-term consequences of menopause. One explanation for this is that they are reluctant to embark on a long-term course of prescription medication, the rationale for which has not been fully described and explained. This is particularly true for HT. There are, of course, other reasons for the concern about HT. A doctor may say "hormones" but for many women, the word that echoes around them is "cancer." The fear of cancer is probably the number one reason for resistance to HT. Another reason is weight gain. No matter how much evidence there is to the contrary, word-of-mouth among menopausal women is that estrogens make you fat. Understandably, menopausal women do not want to put up with unpredictable bleeding, an undeniable side effect risk of ET. Unless the risks and benefits are described in a way that is factual and makes sense, women are reluctant to use HT as advised or, for that matter, to even have the prescription filled.

One out of five women has the conviction that menopause is a natural event that should not require any medication, and up to 50% of women believe that menopause can be adequately managed by approaches other than HT. These attitudes are reinforced when a woman who hesitantly starts HT experiences unexpected and unpleasant side effects such as breast tenderness and irregular bleeding.

The fact that doctors attempt to include advice and explanations that are evidence based does not mean that we have closed minds with respect to alternative approaches to caring for health and well-being. We understand that Ayurvedic and Chinese traditional medicine, for example, were practiced long before the advent of modern Western medicine and that these and other ancient healing arts should not be summarily disregarded. I once visited health clinics in China, many of which offered both Western medicine and Chinese traditional medicine. According to my hosts, the treatment success rate for all conditions in each section was about the same.

Menopausal medicine should include a careful review of overall health issues concerning an individual woman, and no area of concern should be disregarded. If a woman complains of shortness of breath, skin changes, or unwanted weight gain, her health care provider should help her get to the bottom of these problems. Smokers should understand the menopause-specific health risks they carry; there are several. The negative effects of smoking cancel out virtually all the beneficial changes in blood lipid patterns associated with HT. Bone mineral density loss in menopause is more severe among smokers than nonsmokers, and smokers derive less benefit from bone-building therapies. Advice on diet and exercise should be included. A calcium-rich diet, vitamin D and calcium supplements, and weight-bearing exercise all significantly reduce bone mineral loss as women grow older. At any age, a woman should understand that it is never too late to adopt these beneficial lifestyles to maintain cardiovascular health and prevent further bone weakening.

Some women believe that herbs are more beneficial than HT and express a preference for natural agents. However, virtually all of the commonly prescribed HT medications have their origin in a natural product. By far the most frequently prescribed estrogen for the menopause is Premarin, a favorite target of nature-preferring critics. Yet, there is nothing less natural about Premarin than there is, for example, about an estrogen derived from pine needles or soy beans. I have heard the comment that Premarin, which is purified from pregnant mare's urine, is natural only if you are a horse. Does that mean that phytoestrogens in tofu are natural only if you are a soybean? Other commonly prescribed HT preparations are derived from yam or other plant-based sterols, which are the precursor products in the manufacture of estrogenic steroids and most progestins.

The U.S. FDA has scrupulously evaluated each prescription product on the market. The contrast between FDA-approved medications and those that are not FDA regulated is worth reviewing in some detail. For FDA approval, effectiveness has to have been confirmed for each claim in any literature describing the product. This means that you have assurance that the manufacturer's description of the product has been substantiated in studies that have been carefully reviewed and published in the medical literature. As data-based information on a drug's effectiveness, as well as side effects, is collected, it must be transmitted to the FDA where the data are assessed and evaluated. Before the manufacturer can make claims of effectiveness in treating specific symptoms, carefully designed, prospective trials are required. Unless scientifically substantiated, the manufacturer is not permitted to claim effectiveness in its advertising and marketing. For example, the effectiveness of a hormone treatment with regard to controlling hot flashes, other symptoms of vasomotor instability, or vaginal dryness must have been established in properly conducted clinical trials before statements on these issues are allowed. Clinical trial sites are periodically visited and reviewed by FDA monitors. Furthermore, the company is required to list any side effects and adverse reactions to the product. All of this information is summarized in the package insert which accompanies the prescription drug, and it is also listed in an annually updated volume, the *Physicians' Desk Reference*, describing all of the FDA-approved pharmaceuticals. In advertisements published in medical journals, risks and side effects must be included. Moreover, each FDA-approved product must be continuously monitored in a system of postmarketing surveillance designed to uncover any previously unsuspected or unanticipated side effects. This extensive evaluation and surveillance system is designed to protect the public against false claims and misleading advertising as well as to provide an early warning system if problems arise. Even small changes in the incidence of rare events are monitored.

The U.S. drug regulatory system is the world's most stringent, but there is a loophole. Certain products that are described as "naturally occurring" can be marketed as a "dietary supplement" if the manufacturer does not claim that it treats, cures, or prevents a disease. The consumer has no protection under federal law. A company manufacturing such supplements is not required to prove that they are either safe or effective, or even that they work as advertised before they are marketed. When there are serious side effects, they may not be uncovered until large numbers of persons are injured, sometimes seriously.

An example was the discovery of severe liver problems after the use of the dietary herbal supplement kava. Investigative reporters in Europe uncovered some cases that required extreme life-saving measures, such as liver transplants. Although the manufacturer claimed that in many of these cases the patient already had intrinsic liver disease from either alcoholism or hepatitis, sufficient numbers surfaced as to prompt coverage in the press. A report of these cases never appeared in the medical literature so that doctors around the world could not be informed of this serious problem.

Kava is a member of the pepper family and is derived from the root of a tropical plant. It is promoted for the treatment of insomnia and anxiety and has become increasingly popular in Europe, where its main use is for symptoms of depression. In some U.S. health food stores, kava is also sold to manage menopausal symptoms. These claims have never been substantiated.

Another recent example is a modified citrus pectin called PCSPES, promoted for the treatment of prostatic problems, including prostatic cancer. In FDA-sponsored studies, this preparation has been found to be contaminated with warfarin, a commonly prescribed blood thinner known also as coumadin. In California where PCSPES is manufactured, a consumer warning has been issued on the state's medical monitoring web site. Although the manufacturer has now withdrawn PCSPES, bleeding problems causing significant damage may have resulted. This could occur because the manufacturing facilities of nutritional supplements are not subject to inspection and quality control so that pills on the market could be tainted or possibly not produced uniformly. In one study done by the California Department of Health Services, roughly one-third of the

Table 8.1. Herbs Commonly Recommended for Menopause

Common name	Comments
Angelica	No Western medical literature
Black cohosh	Studies available; acts as weak estrogen
Blue cohosh	Nicotinelike; potentially toxic
Chasteberry	No studies; claimed antiandrogen properties
Damiana	No studies; claimed as aphrodisiac
Dong quai, dang gui	Ineffective; potential toxicity
Evening primrose	No benefits over placebo
Ginseng	Claimed as aphrodisiac and alleviating female disorders
Licorice	No studies; potential toxicity
Red clover	Estrogenic; potential toxicity
Saw palmetto	No evidence; may be antiandrogen
St. John's wort	Serotonin inhibitor; potential for drug interaction

Adapted from M. Taylor (1998).

Asian patent medicines that were chemically analyzed were contaminated with heavy metals or pharmaceuticals not listed on the label. Many of these contained more than one contaminant.

Some manufacturers of nutritional supplements have made an effort to provide and maintain a uniform product. They provide data for the U.S. Pharmacopoeia describing their quality control procedures. When verified, the company is entitled to include USP on their labels. Look for this if you intend to take a medication for any purpose. The dosage taken should never exceed 100% of the recommended allowance of any dietary supplement unless there is medical supervision. One reason for this is the possibility of drug interaction with other medications you may be taking.

Table 8.1 lists commonly used food supplements recommended for alleviating menopausal symptoms. More detail about their effectiveness as well as side effects and interactions is included in the subsequent pages. Table 8.1 is a partial list but it includes most of the commonly used preparations.

Black cohosh is known by a variety of other names including black snakeroot, rattle weed, bugwort, and bugbane. It is derived from the rhizomes and roots of the plant. Its active ingredient has been shown to bind to the estrogen receptor in animals and also in women, so it has the biological potential to exert estrogenic action. An alcoholic extract of black cohosh is marketed as Remifemin and is recommended for "female disorders." This terminology is reminiscent of grandma's

Lydia Pinkham's Vegetable Compound that contained black cohosh as its main ingredient.

GlaxoSmithKline, the world's second largest pharmaceutical company, markets Remifemin on all continents. It is sold over the counter in many European countries as well as in the United States and Canada. There are numerous publications on this product which support the claim that it can reduce the number of episodes of vasomotor instability (hot flashes). Hot flashes are caused by the sudden dilation of small blood vessels in the skin, a reaction believed to be a result of low estrogen levels. A product with estrogenic activity, therefore, could ameliorate this symptom. However, the overall effect of the black cohosh product on hormonal status of women has been evaluated with no demonstrable effect on most of the endocrine factors usually influenced by estrogens. One factor, the pituitary's luteinizing hormone, was initially reported to be suppressed, but this has not been confirmed in later studies. In some studies, change has been noted on other estrogen end points such as vaginal maturation or endometrial thickness. Hence, although black cohosh is believed to be estrogenic, there is scant evidence of this when it is subjected to usual measures of estrogenicity. The literature on its effectiveness in reducing menopausal symptoms is based on subjective reports of users. These show significant reduction in number of hot flashes per day, compared to placebo users, and improvement in an index scale that measures a woman's self-evaluation of how she feels (the Kupperman index).

Ginseng has been marketed as an aphrodisiac and also as an agent for amelioration of menopausal symptoms. In a placebo-controlled trial involving nearly 400 postmenopausal women, ginseng caused no reduction in vasomotor symptoms. There was some improvement in depression rates and in vague end points such as general well-being. Ginseng had no estrogenic effect on end organs, such as the vagina, and does not alter pituitary hormone levels, a usual end point to measure estrogenicity. There are no independent studies allowing a determination as to whether ginseng is beneficial.

Dong quai, a Chinese herbal remedy, has been promoted as a "menopausal herb" but has not proved effective in prospective, placebo-controlled studies, in which one group of women is given placebo pills and the other group receives the remedy being tested. Neither the investigators nor the women know which is which. At the end of a specified time period, the results for each group are recorded and compared. This is called a double-blind, prospective study. The measurements included thickness of the endometrium, vaginal maturation (as a measure of improving vaginal dryness), and the subjective reporting of relief of menopausal symptoms. In the study, some coumadinlike action was uncovered, leading to the possibility that the product, especially in excess, could cause serious problems with clotting mechanisms.

An Indian spice, chasteberry, has been marketed for vaginal dryness, low libido, and depression. These are good markers of menopausal changes. Its active ingredient has been shown to bind to the androgen receptor in laboratory studies, but little more is known concerning its clinical effectiveness or side effects.

Since both black cohosh and chasteberry have the potential to modify hormone receptors, as shown in laboratory studies, their use as dietary supplements in menopausal management carries the risk of unexpected hormonal responses; they require more detailed and scientific evaluation.

Evening primrose, also called evening star, is rich in gamma-linolenic acid (GLA) and contains several anticoagulant substances that act like the blood thinner coumadin. For women, evening primrose is commonly recommended for breast pain or breast engorgement, but it is also heavily promoted for menopausal symptoms. The similarity of its richness in GLA to breast milk has led to sweeping claims, never verified, of many health benefits. One positive result was the finding that GLA was effective in treating migraine, but the uncontrolled study design leaves open the question of its validity. GLA is even less well-studied than the other herbal products. The one double-blind study of GLA-rich evening primrose oil led the author to conclude that the GLA offered no benefits over placebo.

A very popular herb used for improvement of overall well being is gingko. It is proposed for the treatment of vascular disorders, memory problems, and neurologic disorders. Ginkgo is of questionable use for memory loss but has some effect on dementia. It is promoted also for relief of menopausal symptoms. In one survey, 16% of menopausal women who used dietary supplements chose gingko. It is claimed that more than 40 double-blind studies demonstrate its benefits, but we have not been able to verify this. With respect to menopausal symptoms, there is no scientific evidence of effectiveness. Gingko, too, has been shown to inhibit platelet-activating factors involved in clotting and among women who are taking anticoagulants for medical reasons has the potential for accentuating the effect of those anticoagulant drugs and hence of producing significant harm.

Licorice, derived from the root of a leguminous plant, has been recommended for menopausal symptoms. Licorice candy contains no actual licorice, but the herbal extract product is used to sweeten cigarettes. Licorice seems to have some estrogenic activity, but its effectiveness has not been confirmed. In large amounts it is associated with disturbances in the levels of both sodium and potassium in the blood.

Red clover, also recommended for the management of menopausal symptoms (broadly defined), has been shown to be clearly estrogenic. Sheep grazing on it have become sterile, suggesting that, at the very least it should be used with extreme caution.

St. John's wort is a commonly used product that has been recommended as an antidepressant as well as an appetite suppressor. The active ingredient of St. John's wort has been identified, and it has been shown in scientific studies to act on the central nervous system as a serotonin reuptake inhibitor. In other words, it modifies the metabolism of the brain in such a way as to reduce depression. The potency of the St. John's wort preparations available over the counter varies. Care with its use is advised because it has been shown to interact adversely with medications used in the management of cardiovascular disease.

A growing number of health care providers incorporate alternative and supplementary modalities in their approach to menopausal medicine. Although much of the information about supplements is passed-down wisdom without verification (some might be in the category referred to disparagingly as "old wives tales"), herbal treatments are certainly suitable for menopausal women who find that these products give them the relief they seek and those who will not or should not use conventional HT for whatever reason. In almost every controlled study of HT there is a demonstrable placebo effect, at least initially. This points out the critical importance of controlled studies in the evaluation of agents used for symptom relief. Most of the herbal medicines are not free of adverse effects, however, so the risk–benefit assessments are generally not completely reliable.

9 • Can phytoestrogens, antioxidants, and vitamins replace HT?

Phytoestrogens, antioxidants, and vitamins are not unfamiliar topics in the discussion of menopause. Among the many alternatives to HT that women lean toward or for which they seek guidance, the most popular are phytoestrogens: soy estrogens in particular. The appeal is understandable since the highly touted benefits claimed for phytoestrogen products sound like all the advantages that scientists are trying to achieve by developing designer estrogens. This multibillion-dollar research effort, supported by federal grants and pharmaceutical company research budgets, is trying to find or develop compounds that retain the benefits of estrogens for the menopausal woman while minimizing or eliminating the risk. New advances are emerging continuously. Now in advanced clinical trials (placebo-controlled, double-blind, prospective studies) are new designer estrogens that protect bone mineral density, improve the blood lipid profile (good cholesterol vs. bad cholesterol), do not stimulate the endometrium, and provide full antagonism of estrogens in breast cancer models. At last two of them are racing to the finish line after hundreds of millions of dollars of research investment and careful FDA scrutiny. In all likelihood, both will soon be available on the prescription drug market.

Save your money, the advocates or distributors of phytoestrogens advise. Nature has already done it for us, and the products are natural. The message seems to be why take "artificial" estrogens when nature has provided a model alternative. Unfortunately, there are scant data to evaluate if these breathtaking claims are valid. Much of the information as to how natural phytoestrogens differ from other estrogens is anecdotal. And the claimants don't have to worry about the FDA looking over their shoulder. Their products are classified as nutritional supplements, not prescription drugs.

Phytoestrogens are exactly what the name implies: They are estrogens that are found in plants. Unless and until we are able to evaluate information about how they differ from other estrogens when they act in the human body, we have to assume that they are no better or worse than other estrogens used in prescription drugs. When there is inadequate published scientific information about them available, compared to the volumes of carefully designed studies required for FDA approval, you have to rely on unsubstantiated claims to decide. It may be useful to make a comparison of data requirements between an FDA-approved prescription drug and a nutritional supplement. Nowadays, a sponsoring company can submit information to the FDA electronically, but if everything required is printed out, the documents and data printouts could fill a small moving van. A diet supplement company planning to market a phytoestrogen can send a letter with a 37-cent stamp.

Soybeans are a very rich source of phytoestrogens. Scientists have discovered the natural occurrence of nonsteroidal phytoestrogens, chiefly isoflavones, in many plants, including grains. Soybeans contain 1–3 mg phytoestrogens per gram of soy protein. That is a remarkable quantity, and the potential for a great deal of estrogen activity.

It raises a puzzling uncertainty about soy estrogens. Ingesting a foodstuff with that amount of isoflavones should result in significant estrogen exposure. Any estrogen target tissue could be inadvertently stimulated. Because tissues of the reproductive system have abundant estrogen receptors, they should be particularly vulnerable. Yet, it is not unusual in pediatric practice to recommend that infants who experience frequent paroxysms of crying or apparent discomfort should be switched from breast milk or conventional dairy-based nutritional formula to soy-based formula The immature human reproductive tract is extremely estrogen sensitive (remember the diethylstilbestrol tragedy in the 1950s). It defies endocrinological logic that in pediatrics, when children are switched to soy-protein formula and are exposed to high doses of soy phytoestrogens, no adverse effects or stimulation of the reproductive tract are reported, but in menopause therapy, soy estrogens are believed to selectively interact with estrogen receptors, including the vaginal mucosa. Reports that soy estrogens restore vaginal moisture in postmenopausal women bring this paradox to mind. Perhaps it is a question of dose differences.

The phytoestrogens, also called isoflavones, extracted from soybeans, include genistein and glycitein. In the past, they have been defined as weak estrogens because they bind much less efficiently to the estrogen receptor than does estradiol. Recall that the receptor is the structure in the cell that recognizes and binds to a circulating hormone. When estrogen and the receptor which recognizes it combine, this estrogen–receptor complex causes the cell to respond. Recent studies have uncovered that the phytoestrogens have a high relative affinity for one of the estrogen receptor subgroups, estrogen receptor beta, than to its counterpart, estrogen receptor alpha. Since the ratio of the two receptors varies from one tissue to another, this makes it possible that the active isoflavone, genistein, would cause a greater response in some tissues than in others. It is believed that this is why they have no effect on the endometrium, and a questionable effect on the breast, a beneficial quality for a menopause treatment. Also beneficial is that they share the characteristics of other estrogens with regard to a heart-friendly effect on lipoproteins. A recent study, however, throws into doubt whether estrogen's beneficial effect on the lipid profile provides the protection for the cardiovascular system that has been assumed.

Interest in the soy phytoestrogens has been sparked by epidemiologic studies on menopausal symptoms and dietary habits in different populations. For example, in parts of the world such as China and Singapore where the diet is rich in soybean phytoestrogens, the incidence of hot flashes is substantially lower than in the European population: as low as 20% as opposed to 80%. These observations have prompted a placebo-controlled study on the impact of soy on hot flashes, and a positive effect on vasomotor symptoms has been reported. Indeed, in one placebo-controlled study there was a definite, statistically significant reduction in the number of hot flashes experienced by the group treated with the soy product. With regard to the effect of soy phytoestrogens on bone loss, there is also promising evidence. A study in China found that bone mineral density values at both the hip and spine region is higher in menopausal women with habitually high intake of dietary isoflavone (from soybean foodstuff such as tofu). The Chinese author was enthusiastic and believes that eating the equivalent of about two pieces of tofu a day can help prevent the onset of osteoporosis.

A double-blind, placebo controlled study in Brazil evaluated the effect of isoflavone on menopausal symptoms. The results indicated a significant decrease in total cholesterol and low-density lipoprotein levels in the isoflavone group. This suggests that isoflavone at a dose of 100 mg daily may be a safe and effective alternative therapy for menopausal symptoms while offering some benefit to the cardiovascular system.

In a recent comprehensive review, U.S. authors point out that the isoflavones that are available as nutritional supplements are only partially purified mixtures and with few exceptions are not rigorously prepared or standardized. They advise that the only satisfactory means of evaluation of the clinical effect of phytoestrogens is to perform well-designed, controlled studies that are carefully monitored. Controlled studies that are available suggest only a modest reduction in menopausal vasomotor symptoms with the use of soy estrogens. In a six-month controlled study, menopausal women ingesting soy estrogens had a dose-dependent increase in the bone density of the spine but not of the hip. At present, no evidence on fracture rates is available, but it is known that a 10% reduction in bone mineral density is associated with a twofold increase in fracture risk. Some scientists believe that there may be a difference in the effectiveness of soy isoflavones contained in the natural foodstuff where they originate and the extracted concentrates used in pill form.

A number of studies have been reported to assess the impact of soy protein on hot flashes. In one Italian study, a 45% reduction in hot flashes was observed as compared with 30% reduction in the placebo-control group. However, compliance was a problem in both groups, and there was a significant dropout rate because of a high incidence of gastrointestinal side effects with the amount of soy protein intake employed in the project. In another study of hot flashes among breast cancer survivors who required an alternative to HT or ET, a formulated soy product was used in a total daily dose of 150 mg isoflavones. Even at this high dose the soy product was not more effective than placebo in reducing vasomotor symptoms.

Some doctors believe that soy estrogen benefits are dose dependent and that studies with ambiguous results do not use high enough doses. Obviously this can be a problem in dietary studies versus those using medication. It has been suggested that most American studies have been done with portions of soy protein per day that are near or below the critical amount needed to get any noticeable effect on menopausal symptoms. The Japanese consume an average of 100–200 mg of soy isoflavones per day, while Americans find it hard to ingest a daily diet with less than half that amount. As much as we enjoy tofu and Japanese dishes, we don't know how to get around this problem.

We conclude that the phytoestrogens are neither sufficiently active nor specific enough to be counted on as sole agents in the management of menopausal symptoms. Available evidence at this time does not support the substitution of soy phytoestrogens for clinically proven methods to manage menopausal symptoms or for the prevention of bone loss in menopausal women. Based on what we now know, they might offer some adjuvant advantage in combination with prescribed estrogen, but well-designed clinical trials are needed to settle some of these important points.

The antioxidants, vitamin C, vitamin E, selenium, and beta carotene, have been marketed as useful in overall preservation of general health and especially in the prevention of chronic disease and cancer. Vitamin E has been suggested for the management of hot flashes. It has been studied in a group of breast cancer survivors, displaying only marginal clinical benefit. Antioxidants are said to work through the protection of the DNA of the vital organ tissues. Their use is widespread, but claims are so generalized that it is difficult to establish effectiveness. Even in randomized, placebo-controlled studies, there is always a significant placebo effect, at least initially. In other words, just taking an inactive pill makes some people report that they are feeling better. For the evaluation of agents used against menopausal symptoms, placebo-controlled studies are critically important. Without them, there can be a lot of wishful thinking. Long-term effects, specifically in the prevention of osteoporosis, are more easily assessed because there are objective measurements of bone density.

We do not agree with the trend to casually experiment with herbs, phytoestrogens, or mega-vitamins. While it is true they probably can't do much harm, by the same token they may not do much good. The most we know about many of them is that they can cause dangerous drug interactions. Someone using a baby aspirin every day to prevent clots or the stronger blood thinner wafarin should not take the risk of increasing blood clotting time even further. Furthermore, the months or years spent on experimenting that will likely lead nowhere would be better spent starting the process of adapting a prescribed HT tailored to individual needs.

10 • Sex and the aging woman

Menopause is looked upon by most women as a clearly identifiable change in their reproductive systems. As the menstrual pattern is altered and menstruation finally ceases, this is a concrete signal that the reproductive tract is changed. In some cases, this is accompanied by decreasing interest in sex, often amounting to complete lack of desire. The cells of the vagina, vulva, and urethra contain a high concentration of estrogen receptors and are especially vulnerable to estrogen deficiency. The net result, without HT/ET, is a dramatic anatomical change in these organs. In the absence of estrogen support, the vaginal tissues gradually become thin and lose their tone and elasticity. The fluid which normally is released across the vaginal lining during sexual excitement is reduced. The famous sexology team William Masters and Virginia Johnson actually filmed this fluid release during sexual stimulation. I was present when they showed this film to professional colleagues for the first time. The distinguished professor of gynecology Alan Guttmacher was in the small audience. When the film was over he declared with genuine enthusiasm, "I have been doing pelvic examinations throughout my career and never thought we would ever see such convincing and direct evidence of the changes in the vagina that occur during excitation." Another distinguished professor of gynecology left the room without saying a word. From the grim look of disapproval on his face I would guess that sexual aspects of the menopause were not part of the residency training program at his medical center.

Estrogen deprivation results in decreased or even absent lubrication so that intercourse becomes unpleasant or even painful. Understandably such changes contribute greatly to the lack of interest in sex. By no means do all menopausal women experience these symptoms. Especially vulnerable, however, are those whose sexual relationships have been altered by divorce, separation, or illness or those whose husbands have lost sex interest. Women who have experienced satisfying sex during their reproductive lives are better able to cope with menopausal alterations. A Swedish survey found that 70% of women 46 years of age reported that they continued to function sexually. In a group of 62-year-old women, this declined to 39%. In about half the cases the lack of a regular sex life was attributed to absence of a partner or lack of a partner's desire. Social factors have a major impact on sexual patterns, but they are not the whole story. Many women make a conscious decision not to have intercourse because of either lack of desire on their part or pain. This is especially common in the older age group who are not using ET/HT.

There is a clear link, shown by scientific studies, between menopausal vaginal symptoms and decreased sexual activity. In research of this type, sexual function is evaluated subjectively using a detailed questionnaire. One study reported that about 20% of premenopausal women reported less than ideal vaginal lubrication. This dropped to about 14% in the perimenopausal age group but increased to 44% in postmenopausal women. A similar trend is reported for pain with intercourse ("dyspareunia"). Dyspareunia was reported by 10% of premenopausal women, 7% of perimenopausal women, and 20% of postmenopausal women. All of these changes are associated with decreased levels of sex-related activities. In postmenopausal women as compared with premenopausal women, there is a reduced amount of petting and foreplay and lower frequency of intercourse, masturbation, and sexual fantasy.

Sexual function is often ignored during doctor visits, even when the doctor has been through a residency program in gynecology. The sexual component of the reproductive system has not been sufficiently stressed as an important life factor in medical evaluation generally. In a 2001 review of the status of postmenopausal therapy in the *New England Journal of Medicine*, sexual function is not mentioned at all. As a gynecologist, it has been my experience that the subject is usually not raised spontaneously by menopausal women during the annual checkup. It doesn't take long to address this area, and just as one would routinely review other bodily functions, sexual matters should be discussed. I usually start by asking whether there is any pain with intercourse or problems with lubrication. Sometimes the response is, "We are not having any intercourse because of my husband's 'problem'." The response is undoubtedly accurate in many cases, but I can sometimes tell that it is a polite way of closing the door on the subject. Women seem to have been conditioned, perhaps by society's mores, to avoid talking about these issues, even with their gynecologist. In these days erectile function is discussed freely and openly in television ads for Viagra, but there are no similar advertisements for treatment of lubrication problems and sexual response in women.

When sex is discussed, the typical complaint is vaginal dryness. This serves as a signal to the doctor to explore sexual matters further. Is it that the patient has the sensation that the vulvar and vaginal area are dry, or is she referring specifically to the lubrication which occurs during sexual arousal? Is she experiencing slow or even absent response to sexual stimulation? Has this subject come up in conversations with her partner? Have relationships between the two been altered in nonsexual spheres? Do these perceived physical changes lead to avoidance of intercourse, or is it that there is no physical desire even to initiate sexual communication? Is there failure to respond sexually even though positively disposed? If there is decreased lubrication, has this affected ability to achieve orgasm? Is there actual pain on penetration? Has there been a change during self-stimulation? The overall picture can help decide among the various approaches to treatment that might best be tried—ET with or without testosterone, local estrogen therapy, simple lubrication, further counseling, or some combination of these.

It is helpful to understand changes that occur during the normal process of sexual arousal, knowledge gleaned by the early studies of Masters and Johnson. Arousal initiates an increase in blood flow to the genital area. This leads to congestion of the veins (vasocongestion) in the vulvar and clitoral area and a release of lubricating moisture across the vaginal wall. The clitoris distends and the vagina and vulva become moist and warm as a result. These changes are influenced by the woman's hormones, and estrogen plays a major part. One solution when there is a problem is local or systemic estrogen replacement. Under the influence of ET/HT, the vaginal wall begins to thicken within a matter of days and the lubricating function begins to return.

What about the woman who cannot or should not take estrogen because of clear-cut contraindications or because she prefers not to take hormones? A variety of alternative options are available. The most obvious of these is the use of a lubricant during intercourse. Vaseline is messy and is not recommended. A water-soluble lubricant, such as KY Jelly, can be used, but it also tends to be messy. Several over-the-counter preparations (e.g., Astroglide) designed to mimic the lubricant which normally appears in the vagina are available and are very effective in this regard. A moisturizing vaginal suppository, marketed as Replens, can be inserted daily as needed to produce a continuous moisturizing effect.

Women who have had an entirely satisfactory sex life before menopause are much more likely to maintain sexual function afterward. Intercourse itself, perhaps with the help of a vaginal lubricant, will go far in maintaining the elasticity and receptivity of the vaginal area. Estrogen-containing vaginal cream applied twice weekly produces a significant local effect on the vagina while causing only a minor rise in circulating estrogen. A vaginal estrogen tablet, marketed as Vagifem, has been studied extensively. Tablets are introduced into the vagina, where they are slowly absorbed, providing direct contact of the estrogen with the vaginal epithelial lining and producing an excellent local effect with minimal systemic absorption. In Brazil, Elsimar Coutinho has for many years advocated the use of vaginal pills for the administration of reproductive hormones (even for contraception) and usually recommends this as an initial approach for his menopausal patients with vaginal symptoms. Also available is an estrogen-releasing vaginal ring (Estring) or vaginal creams (Estrace, Premarin, Ortho Dienestrol). Vaginal estrogens offer an alternative for women for whom systemic estrogen treatment is ill advised on medical grounds.

Although the physical changes that occur in the vulvar and vaginal regions contribute to sexual dysfunction in menopause, the central nervous system is also involved. Contributing psychological factors are complex and can be assessed objectively only with great difficulty. As some areas of the central nervous system contain estrogen receptors, it is not surprising that estrogen has a direct influence on the central nervous system. This observation prompted numerous investigations to explore a link between bioavailable estrogen levels and central nervous system function. Estrogen, for example, lowers the levels of a key enzyme (monoamine oxidase, MAO) that is involved in synthesis and metabolism of serotonin, a chemical messenger of the central nervous system. When MAO is reduced, there is a higher level of serotonin, a factor important in the prevention of depression. Because of this effect on MAO and serotonin, mood is positively affected by estrogen. Estrogen deprivation can lead to increased irritability and depression.

Testosterone production in women is normal; both the ovaries and the adrenals produce testosterone. Androgens are present in about equal amounts in both males and females, and circulating androgens are present in much higher concentrations than estrogens in both men and women. In women, much of the androgen that is produced is converted to estrogen before it exerts its effect, but every woman is left with a significant androgen concentration. Testosterone can act directly on the brain, and there are androgen receptors in both the central nervous system and the genital tissues of both sexes.

Many studies reveal that the ovaries continue to produce androgens after menopause, but the androgen that has received the most attention is produced both by the ovaries and by the adrenal gland. This is DHEA (dehydroepiandrosterone) and its counterpart, DHEAS (dehydroepiandrosterone sulfate). DHEAS has been referred to as a spring board hormone for female sexuality, and efforts have been made to assess its role in sexual function. Levels of DHEAS begin to appear at about age 10, peak at age 20, and then gradually regress.

The role of DHEAS in sexual function has recently been reassessed in women with clinically established adrenal insufficiency. In these women who have low levels of DHEAS, a dramatic improvement in libido and sexual responsiveness has been reported after replacement therapy using oral doses of DHEA. This observation is used as justification for menopausal women taking DHEA to improve libido. There are conflicting studies, however. In untreated Australian women, ages 45–55, it was found that sexual dysfunction increases rather sharply from about 40% to close to 90% from early to late in the menopausal transition. This change in sexual function is correlated with decreasing circulating estrogen levels, but not with alterations in DHEA or testosterone levels. It is suggested, based on these observations, that the decline in sexual function is related almost exclusively to estrogen. This study fails to support the observation that androgens positively affect sexual function.

Nevertheless, DHEA has been promoted to treat the menopausal symptoms attributed to androgen deficiency and is available in various preparations in health food stores. The significant placebo impact associated with the evaluation of agents designed to improve well-being and sexual function needs to be carefully considered. At least one controlled, prospective study failed to establish the effectiveness of DHEA. In the laboratory, studies have found that tissues obtained from postmenopausal ovaries can continue to produce androgen, but other studies have failed to confirm these findings.

A commonly used clinical approach is to combine small amounts of testosterone with the estrogen in the HT regimen. A combination product is available which in controlled trials was shown to be associated with enhanced psychological well being as well as sexual desire in addition to increased frequency of intercourse and orgasm, as compared with women who were treated with estrogen alone. The downside to the use of testosterone is facial hair growth. At a dose of 150 mg of testosterone per day, this side effect is noted in as many as 20% of women. A lower dose, however, decreases the incidence of hirsutism drastically, to less than 5%. The commercially available product (Estratest) contains 2.5 mg or 1.25 mg of methyltestosterone in each tablet. The addition of the methyl group to the testosterone molecule significantly increases its potency and effectiveness when taken orally. There is certainly a variable response to testosterone from one woman to the next, and hence the importance of monitoring and adjusting the dose carefully in women who are using this combination. The long-term effect of the estrogen/testosterone combination overall is under continuing surveillance. The changes in serum cholesterol are mixed. A decrease in high-density lipoprotein (HDL), the good cholesterol, is troubling, but there is also a decrease in triglycerides and low-density lipoprotein, making the change in HDL somewhat less worrisome.

The problem with evaluating the impact of any agent on sexual function is that there are many factors to consider in addition to hormonal factors. Women who report a healthy sexual desire before the onset of the perimenopause/menopause but who exhibit a decrease in libido after menopause are most likely to benefit from testosterone. No hormone can solve problems of life's stress, and endocrine manipulation is certainly no panacea when there has been previous sexual dysfunction.

Women who have had surgical removal of both ovaries experience the most abrupt decline in circulating androgen concentrations. This group benefits most reliably from androgen replacement. For some unexplained reason, a lower level of libido and orgasmic response occurs more often in women who have had their ovaries removed but not their uterus compared to those undergoing a hysterectomy with removal of the ovaries. Since the ovaries produce half of a woman's testosterone (the other half comes from the adrenal gland), testosterone levels drop 50% after the ovaries are surgically removed. This is why the changes in the reproductive tract are more dramatic and abrupt in women whose menopause is induced surgically rather than progressively with age, and why adding testosterone to the estrogen replacement in this group is particularly helpful.

A specific syndrome, referred to as "androgen insufficiency syndrome," has been popularized. Its components include a number of symptoms such as decrease in sexual desire or fantasy and low libido. There is also a decreased sense of well-being and unexplained fatigue. Because these are subjective symptoms without measurable parameters, the syndrome remains vague and ill defined. The medical conditions associated with androgen insufficiency syndrome include premature ovarian failure, adrenal insufficiency, impaired function of the pituitary gland, and glucocorticoid therapy which alters adrenal function. After androgen treatment, women with these conditions report improvement in sexual desire and activity and increased sexual responsiveness and orgasm. Whether it is an actual benefit of the treatment or a placebo response, the feeling that a treatment is working is especially important when the end point is one or another aspect of sexuality.

Testosterone can be taken orally, but it is absorbed more efficiently from transdermal patches or by creams or gels. It is also available by injection or subcutaneous implants. A woman using testosterone should be conscientious about following up with medical monitoring for signs of virilization such as acne, hirsutism, fluid retention, and excessive production of red cells. Some doctors (usually male) show undue concern about "aggressive behavior" when women are on testosterone supplementation therapy, but this is not one of the side effects noted in clinical trials.

11 • What is the status of designer estrogens?

The choice of any medication depends on the balance of the risks and the benefits. This is the critical factor in choosing hormone therapy. It is the motivation behind the search for specially designed molecules that could prevent the symptoms associated with decreased production of estrogen such as hot flashes, vaginal dryness, and other issues which may be estrogen-related, including sleep disturbances and memory loss, while at the same time protecting both the bones and the cardiovascular system well into old age. Moreover, the goal is to achieve all of this without any short-term or long-term adverse effects on the breast, uterus, and cardiovascular or clotting systems.

The age of modern molecular biology has brought to the fore a field that is not as well known in the public media as exciting subjects like the human genome or stem cell research. This is the field of receptor biology. It has clarified how hormones work and has helped identify medications that can preferentially affect some organ systems but not others. In the case of estrogen action, such agents are referred to as selective estrogen receptor modulators (SERMs.) They exert their effect selectively at the cellular level by modulating the estrogen receptors that determine whether and how strongly a tissue responds to estrogen stimulation. An ideal SERM would preferentially affect the bones positively, preventing osteoporosis while controlling the common menopausal symptoms such as hot flashes and vaginal dryness associated with the vaginal atrophy, while also having a positive effect on circulating lipids and cardiovascular system. It should be able to do all of this without any effect on the breast or the uterine lining.

Estrogens have the potential for causing cell proliferation in the uterine lining (endometrium) and in the cells of the breast ducts and lobules. Constant stimulation of the endometrium by "unopposed" estrogen can lead to precancerous changes and even frank carcinoma. This is why estrogens cannot be used alone in women with a uterus, and the typical menopausal hormone therapy includes a progestin to prevent this complication. Adding a progestin, however, does not protect the cells of the breast from estrogen stimulation, so that some increase in the risk of breast cancer during long-term therapy use remains.

No ideal SERM has yet been developed, but SERMs are available that do not cause proliferation of breast cells while maintaining bone strength and decreasing the incidence of bone fracture. One such agent is tamoxifen, marketed as Nolvadex, and another is raloxifene, marketed as Evista.

Tamoxifen was developed as an antiestrogen, a compound with the ability to block the action of estrogens. When we collaborated to study a related compound, known as MRL-41, we showed that it was an antiestrogen that also acted as a weak estrogen. That was before the revolution in receptor biology, so we were not able to recognize the potential of that type of compound for hormone therapy. MRL-41 and its counterpart, clomiphene citrate, had a surprising and unexpected action. In women who were infertile because they had stopped ovulating, clomiphene citrate induced them to ovulate, and, in many cases, pregnancy followed. The mechanism behind this was not worked out until much later, when it was discovered that clomiphene citrate functioned as a SERM. It is estrogenic in that it triggers the release of pituitary hormones, which stimulate the ovaries to ovulate while at the same time having virtually no effect on other estrogen-sensitive tissues.

Tamoxifen was introduced for the treatment of breast cancer when its estrogen-receptor–modifying activity was discovered and early clinical trials showed that it was an effective treatment. Current practice calls for the use of tamoxifen for five years in node-positive as well as node-negative breast cancers which contain the estrogen-receptor positivity. Its effectiveness is now well established. The primary FDA-approved indication for tamoxifen is for the treatment of diagnosed breast cancer. Approval has been extended for breast cancer prevention in women with a high-risk of breast cancer (smokers with a strong family history of the disease, for example.)

During the clinical trials of tamoxifen, it was discovered that the drug prevents bone loss. In other words, tamoxifen has an effect on the bones similar to that of estrogen. At the same time, its effect on the breast is antiestrogenic. In addition to its beneficial effect on bone and breast cells, tamoxifen lowers circulating cholesterol. This suggests that it may be useful in preventing or retarding the progression of coronary heart disease but this remains unproven. Much like clomiphene citrate, it can induce ovulation in women who are not ovulating.

In spite of these positive attributes, undesirable tamoxifen side effects reduce its usefulness for HT in women who are otherwise healthy. Tamoxifen not only fails to prevent hot flashes, but it usually accentuates their intensity and duration. This is a result of its antiestrogenic action. The vasomotor instability associated with tamoxifen use is sometimes debilitating, but women who are being treated for breast cancer have a substantial motivation for continuing treatment in spite of these side effects. Tamoxifen may also increase the risk of blood clots and thromboembolic disease. Its estrogenic property stimulates growth of the endometrium, so it is associated with an increased risk of endometrial polyps and endometrial cancer. Women who are receiving tamoxifen alone must be monitored carefully because endometrial hyperplasia or even cancer can be diagnosed in its early stages. This complication is markedly reduced in estrogen-treated women by the addition of a progestin.

Raloxifene (Evista) has become an important alternative in menopausal management. The FDA has approved raloxifene for the treatment and prevention of osteoporosis in postmenopausal women. It can reduce the risk of vertebral fractures in postmenopausal women by nearly 50%. Like tamoxifen, however, raloxifene does not relieve vasomotor flushes, and it can increase the risk of deep vein thrombosis. Sixty-five to 75% of tamoxifen-treated women experience hot flashes, and in 80% of these, the hot flashes persist for more than one year. Unless a SERM of this type is being used to treat or prevent breast cancer, there is less incentive to continue to use it when hot flashes are markedly exacerbated. Another disadvantage is that raloxifene does not affect the vagina. Hence, the vaginal mucosa continues to become thinner with time. This is associated with vaginal dryness and increased difficulty with penetration during intercourse. This symptom can be managed to a degree, but not entirely, with vaginal lubricants, but it remains a major source of concern in menopausal patients on raloxifene. Similar to tamoxifen and estrogen, raloxifene increases the risk of venous thrombosis.

Like tamoxifen, raloxifene decreases total cholesterol as well as low-density lipoprotein (LDL), the bad cholesterol. Treatment with raloxifene does not appear to change high-density lipoprotein (HDL) cholesterol or triglycerides levels in circulation. Its effect on the breast is of major importance. Studies have now shown that there is a lower risk of breast cancer in raloxifene-treated women, and studies are ongoing to evaluate its effectiveness in reducing breast cancer risk in women who do not have the disease but are considered to be at high risk. It certainly does not harm breast tissue in any way.

In contrast to tamoxifen, raloxifene does not stimulate the endometrium. It increases bone density and lowers cholesterol. It does not have a protective effect on the vagina, and, if anything, exacerbates the severity and frequency of hot flashes.

The clinically important difference between raloxifene and tamoxifen is in the potential for tamoxifen to stimulate endometrial growth. With regard to the effect on the breast, tamoxifen has been shown to decrease the risk of breast cancer in high-risk patients by as much as 45%. This effect has been observed in both pre- and postmenopausal women. Furthermore, tamoxifen prevents the recurrence of breast cancer. Both agents have a positive influence on bones, and both are equally ineffective in addressing the standard symptoms of the menopause such as hot flashes and vaginal dryness. In contrast to standard HT, tamoxifen has not been associated with breast tenderness and discomfort (mastodynia). Mastodynia occurs infrequently in raloxifene-treated patients although it is seen slightly more than in untreated patients. Except for the management of breast cancer, tamoxifen is generally not recommended for menopause.

Raloxifene, on the other hand, presents some advantages because of the absence of stimulation of either the endometrium or the breasts, as well as its prevention of bone mineral density loss and osteoporosis. It is therefore not an unreasonable choice for women with uteri who, during the course of HT, experience breast pain or other side effects that lead to dissatisfaction with the treatment. Raloxifene should also be considered by women who are in the high-risk category for breast cancer or for those who have benign but persistent endometrial bleeding that is not controlled by moderating the dose or method of administration of HT. Its principal drawback, lack of prevention of hot flashes and vaginal atrophy, would make raloxifene a less acceptable method for a woman whose primary concern is these quality-of-life symptoms.

Tibolone is a synthetic steroid that could offer another choice for HT. It is not yet available in the United States but has been used in 60 countries for about a decade. In European countries it is marketed under the trade name Livial. Although its use has been primarily for prevention of osteoporosis, it has characteristics that make it interesting for more general application in menopause. Tibolone affects estrogen receptors, progesterone receptors, and androgen receptors in a selective manner. It has the bone-protective effects of an estrogen and, because of its ability to combine with estrogen receptors, provides relief of hot flashes and vaginal dryness. In one comparative study, tibolone alone was found to be as effective in treating hot flashes and vaginal dryness as a popular combination HT.

Moreover, tibolone and its associated metabolites may protect the breast against estrogenic stimulation. This drug could, therefore, lower the risk of breast cancer. Tibolone's inherent progestational activity suppresses estrogen-induced hyperplasia of the endometrium so that it can be used alone, without the addition of a progestational agent. Many studies have been reported on the safety of this product, and there are plans to introduce it in the United States market once approved by the FDA. Although there are no long-term studies looking at cardiovascular risks, attention will have to be given to its affect on blood lipids because it has been reported to selectively lower HDL cholesterol levels without changing LDL cholesterol levels. This results in an unfavorable shift in the cholesterol ratio. If approved and introduced in the United States, tibolone's particular niche could be for women who do not want to take estrogen or are unwilling to accept the breakthrough bleeding of other HT regimens but who are particularly concerned about bone loss and want to reduce the risk of fractures.

The first and second generation SERMs (tamoxifen and raloxifene) have been successful in treating at least one of the afflictions common among women in the menopause, but they have not been shown to positively affect many of the other symptoms of the menopause such as hot flashes, vaginal dryness, and urinary problems. Since these quality-of-life issues are what prompt most women to seek hormone replacement in the first place, the search for newer SERMs continues. There are other promising SERMs in the research pipelines of major pharmaceutical companies. Starting with a new chemical entity and carrying it through all the required preclinical studies, safety studies, and ultimate development as a new drug can cost $400–$500 million, so usually only the large companies can afford such an investment, and they don't initiate the work casually. Both Pfizer and Wyeth, major pharmaceutical companies with strong research and development programs, have publicly announced their progress with SERMs that may win back women who have discontinued HT out of fear of side effects. They are referred to as third- generation SERMs.

Bazedoxifene is the Wyeth compound. It binds to both types of estrogen receptors and has an array of tissue-specific actions that hold promise for use in HT. It shows no activity when studied in the laboratory using a breast cancer cell proliferation assay. It does not stimulate growth of the endometrium. In animal studies, it lowers total cholesterol. For maintaining bone mineral density and bone strength, it is estimated to be 10-fold more potent than raloxifene. Its main difference (and a significant advantage over their earlier SERMs) is that it does not increase the number of hot flashes.

Since it is being developed by Wyeth, the same company that markets Premarin, bazedoxifene is being tested in combination with that familiar equine estrogen. The combination's performance suggests advantages over the familiar Prempro product; it reduces the number of hot flashes while cutting down on the stimulation of the endometrium. If it meets its potential after extensive clinical evaluation, bazedoxifene with or without Premarin is likely to have a major impact on HT. Final testing and FDA approval may take until 2005.

Lasofoxifene, the Pfizer product under study, has similar advantages to bazedoxifene. Its development may take a shorter time to reach completion. It is a very powerful compound so that benefits are achieved with very low doses. For example, at only 0.25 mg per day, it improves bone mineral density of the lumbar spine to a greater extent than achieved when a woman takes 60 mg per day of raloxifene. At the same dose comparisons, the compound outperforms raloxifene in lowering serum LDL-cholesterol and equals raloxifene in reducing endometrial stimulation. Like bazedoxifene, in laboratory studies it does not appear to stimulate the growth of breast cells.

The great advantage of evidence-based medicine is that evaluations can be made on the basis of established facts and concrete data. Chemists started by constructing molecules specifically designed to modify estrogen receptors, and pharmacologists carried out evaluations that produced results that could be analyzed microscopically as well as by statistical methods. Clinical investigators are now carrying the process to completion under the watchful eye of the FDA. Baby boomers heading past 50 will be the beneficiaries. The options open to them will not be their mothers' HT.

II • • • Male Andropause

12 • Is there a "male menopause"?

Stories about aged fathers are legion, not only in the Bible but also in present times. According to the *Guinness Book of Records*, the oldest natural father in 2000 was Hu Chin-yao of Taiwan at age 109 years. Credibility of such claims aside, the asserted lifetime reproductive potential of the male does not represent a more advanced reproductive system than the female. To the contrary, the male system is an atavistic carryover from our evolutionary past, with striking similarities to a frog, fish, or mouse, whereas adaptations in the female reproductive system provide the evolutionary advances needed for our highly successful process of assuring nurture and support for single newborns.

A microscopist looking at a human testis sees a structure remarkably similar to that of lower vertebrates—a compact body of tightly convoluted tubules held intact by a shiny, fibrous sheath. The structure of the human testis might be characterized as generic. The seminiferous tubules, in which sperm production takes place, would extend for several miles if straightened out. This tubular structure separates the sperm-producing function of the male gonad from the cells that produce its hormones (predominantly testosterone and other androgens). The sperm are produced inside the seminiferous tubules, which make up most of the bulk and weight of the testis, and the hormone-producing cells (Leydig cells) occupy the space outside the tubules. This is an important difference from the follicle of the ovary where egg and hormone production are part of an integrated unit, so when one declines or ends, the other does also.

The testis retains throughout life the ability to make sperm because it never runs out of the primordial cells, spermatogonia, which can divide over and over again. These are the primitive stem cells that can give rise to sperm. The multiplication phase of spermatogonia in the testis is not restricted to fetal life, as is the multiplication phase of oogonia in the ovary of the female. The cell divisions go on and on; no matter how many sperm are produced, there are always more spermatogonia that keep on dividing and produce still more. Consequently, the human male produces countless spermatozoa in a lifetime, a trait reminiscent of species that entrust their survival to the release of copious numbers of sperm in the general surroundings of egg clutches discharged by the female into seawater, tidal marshes, or ponds. For these species, the strategy for reproductive success is the fertilization of multitudes of eggs with the expectation that at least a few offspring will survive.

The man's billions of sperm come from the 1000–2000 primitive stem cells that migrate into the embryonic testis before the end of the second month of intrauterine life and from then on never stop multiplying. Unlike the ovary, which has a limited functional span because of the follicle-depleted mechanism of atresia, the testis has no such mechanism to end the potential of reproduction.

With respect to sperm production, therefore, there is not a male equivalent to the loss of fertility accompanying the onset of menopause. There is no built-in, genetically controlled process of testicular senescence as there is for the ovary. To the contrary, there is a genetically encoded ability to produce sperm throughout life. The hormone-producing capacity of the testis, however, is not as well conserved. In healthy men, bioactive testosterone levels in the blood decline by approximately 1% per year between ages 40 and 70. During this time, the levels drop almost 40%.

There is a natural depletion of the hormone-producing Leydig cells with aging, and this depletion can be caused as a secondary result of other bodily changes that occur with advancing years. Even when sperm production continues, secretion of hormones by the testis can decline. With aging, it is not uncommon for vascular changes to affect the testis, the pituitary, or the brain and indirectly cause a decrease of testicular hormone production. Adult onset diabetes can also disturb nerve or vascular function and interrupt testicular function.

There can be, therefore, a "male menopause" (an inaccurate label) or "andropause," but its cause is quite different from the cause of menopause in women. Andropause is the result of androgen deficiency that is usually a secondary result of other changes in the body, not because the testis reaches a depletion point of no return, as the ovary does in the woman. Doctors who specialize in reproductive medicine do not like the term "male menopause" but they accept "andropause." They prefer to use the descriptive terms "partial androgen deficiency in aging men" (PADAM) or "partial endocrine deficiency in aging men" (PEDAM) because these terms more accurately define the condition. PEDAM is the more comprehensive of the two because it refers not only to the androgen deficiency that can occur with aging, but also to other endocrine factors. Thyroid function and growth hormone production, for example, frequently decline with aging.

A study I did on testicular function in aging confirmed that a number of changes could be ascribed to different causes. About half of men in their 80s still had cells in their testis that retained the capacity to produce steroid hormones, but there was a shift in the ratio of estrogen to androgen found in their blood and urine. Aging brought on a higher proportion of estrogen production or conversion of androgens to estrogen. Some men had testicular atrophy because there was an impairment of the pituitary gland caused by a restriction of its blood supply as a result of arteriosclerosis. The testis depends on pituitary hormone stimulation in order to function. In the absence of these hormonal messages from the pituitary gland, both sperm production and hormone production cease.

Other men in the group studied had an aging change analogous to menopause; the pituitary produces its gonad-stimulating hormone, but the target cells in the testis lose their capacity to respond, so that testicular hormone production is low while the blood level of the pituitary's gonad-stimulating hormone is elevated. The cause for this could be vascular changes around the testis or changing sensitivity of the Leydig cells to the stimulatory effect of pituitary hormones. Still other men in the study, almost one out of five, had hormone and sperm production about the same as much younger men. Unlike its female counterpart, partial androgen deficiency does not affect all aging men. Without a careful endocrinological evaluation, it is not possible to make the distinction. Estimates range from 20% to more than 50% of men over the age of 60 who have significant androgen deficiency.

Understanding the normal function of the testis gives an appreciation of what changes in testicular function mean for a man's health and well-being. Testosterone is the main product of the hormone-producing cells of the testis, but it also produces other androgens and a small quantity of estrogens. So first we have to discard the idea that testosterone and other androgens are exclusively male sex hormones and estrogens are solely female sex hormones. Both are present in men and women. Testosterone can be converted to estrogen in many tissues, including the brain and breast, which is a normal process. The chemical conversion of the testosterone molecule to the estrogen molecule is called aromatization.

Once produced by the Leydig cells of the testis, testosterone can also be converted to androgens of higher potency such as dihydrotestosterone (DHT), which is more than twice as strong as testosterone. This usually occurs in the tissues of the prostate gland, other organs of the male reproductive system, and the skin. Some of the testosterone and other androgens are converted to inactive metabolites and excreted. This conversion takes place primarily in the liver.

Androgens, the predominant products of the Leydig cells, have two classes of activity. They stimulate the sexual characteristics of a man; this is the androgenic action. Equally important, they act on many other tissues, such as muscle, and they have an important influence on general body metabolism. This is called anabolic action because it promotes tissue growth. The opposite action is catabolism, the process of tissue breakdown.

The important role of the androgenic (masculinizing) effects of testosterone can be seen throughout the animal kingdom. Manifestations of these effects range from such majestic ornaments as the antler of the elk or the mane of the lion to the obscure thumb pads of the male frog, seemingly unimpressive but vitally important for clasping the female during the mating season to assure that sperm and eggs find each other. The boar's tusk, the ram's horns, and the rooster's comb and spurs are all masculine characteristics that respond to the action of testosterone. When a young male puppy starts raising his leg instead of squatting, it's because testosterone has kicked in.

In humans, testosterone production begins in the seventh week of fetal life and directs the necessary changes during development to establish the male sex characteristics, even behavioral patterns. There is no doubt that testosterone acts on the brain in the early developmental stages of human life. Without testosterone in these early fetal days, even genetic males would develop female reproductive organs. Late in pregnancy, having made its imprint to assure male differentiation, testosterone declines as the hormone-producing Leydig cells temporarily disappear or become inactive. At puberty, they reawaken. The new surge of testosterone stimulates maturation of the penis, scrotum, prostate, and seminal vesicle. Hair-growth patterns, voice changes, and bone configuration are controlled by testicular androgens. Beginning in adolescence and throughout adult life, they facilitate libido and sexual potency, as well as aggressive behavior. There is hardly an organ that does not respond to androgens in some way. Skin, brain, kidney, muscle, and pituitary are some examples. Androgen receptors within cells or on the cell-surface membrane determine whether they are targets for androgens. These receptors are specialized molecules that can latch on to testosterone as it passes by in the blood and help to select the desired effects that will result from the hormone's stimulation.

With this panoply of activities in mind, it is clear that if androgen levels decline with aging, for whatever reason, major shifts in physical and psychological status can be expected. There is a decrease in muscle strength and a deposition of abdominal fat. Symptoms include loss of muscle and bone mass, lack of energy, loss of balance, increased frailty, and decreased general well-being. The body's ability to respond to infection is reduced. Not only is there a decrease in immune response, but there is also a decline in the concentration of red blood cells, the oxygen-carrying component of the blood. As both the production and availability of biologically active androgens decrease, there is a decrease in libido, sexual potency, and erectile function. Androgen deficiency is associated with an increase in sleep disorders, irritability, and other mood changes. Some claim that it is also linked to memory loss and other cognitive functions. Together, these changes either in total or in part have come to be known as andropause, or androgen deficiency of aging men.

Men produce estrogens that play the same vital role in maintaining bone density that these hormones have in women. If estrogen levels decline in men, there is also a decrease in bone mass with an increased risk of fractures. Estrogens have other functions as well, including a role in regulating how testosterone is managed in the bloodstream and eventually metabolized. When testosterone enters the bloodstream, most of it is bound to a protein that makes the complex water-soluble. Because of its molecular structure, testosterone is mostly insoluble in the blood plasma. In its bound form testosterone is inactive. Only the relatively tiny unbound portion can make its way to target cells and exert its manifold influences. Estrogen in men stimulates the formation of this binding protein by the liver and therefore indirectly causes a reduction of the free, active testosterone. Through this mechanism, when the estrogen level increases with aging, it can have a major influence in causing androgen insufficiency.

There are other changes in the burden of illness of the aging male that are not directly the result of androgen deficiency but which may result from the lifestyle occasioned by the ebb in levels of testicular hormones. When men become less active and more obese, for example, they increase their risk of cardiovascular disease or lung disease, the major causes of death in men over 60.

Androgen decline in the aging male is a fact of life. It leads to a syndrome in aging men consisting of physical, sexual, behavioral, and psychological symptoms that include weakness, fatigue, reduced muscle and bone mass, impaired red blood cell production, reduced or absent sperm production, sexual dysfunction, depression, anxiety, memory impairment, and reduced cognitive function. While the physiological events that cause this change of life are not the same as the reasons for estrogen decline in women, the result is similar to menopause.

Like women's menopause, partial androgen deficiency in the aging male need not be an inevitable consequence of aging. Proper management of lifestyle and androgen supplementation therapy can protect against the changes brought on by androgen deficiency and prevent the onset of frailty in older men.

13 • Is testosterone the only androgen the body produces?

The testis produces several different hormones with androgenic activity. Testosterone is the most well known. It gets blamed for everything macho and its loss is lamented as a farewell to verve. A gradual decline in testosterone begins from the peak blood levels at about 20 years of age. Between ages 50 and 80, the average level of bioavailable testosterone falls more than 50%. There has been an effort to find synthetic compounds that can offset this aging decline. Androgens with unusual chemical structures proved to be a misguided approach because of their association with liver toxicity. Unlike estrogenic hormones, plants and other natural sources have failed to provide a source of androgens for human application. Consequently, the source of molecular models for testosterone substitutes has been the human body.

The normal pathways in the body for the synthesis of testosterone explain why men use various testosterone precursor compounds for bodybuilding or to derive other benefits from higher testosterone levels. Sold as nutritional supplements, these precursors are active orally and can be converted in the body to testosterone. Claims that are made for these products must be evaluated with the realization that they are not regulated by the FDA and manufacturers have to prove neither their claims nor product safety before marketing those supplements.

Testosterone is by far the most abundant androgen in the body, but it is not the most potent. That distinction belongs to dihydrotestosterone, one of the conversion products of testosterone. A testosterone precursor, androstenediol, is also a considerably stronger androgen. It has several isomers, or chemical forms, and these vary in androgenic potency. Two weaker androgens that are rapidly converted to testosterone are DHEA (dehydroepiandrosterone) and its conversion product, androstenediol. If these compounds sound familiar, it may be because you can find an entire shelf devoted to products containing them in nutrition stores. They are also popular subjects of web pages and magazine articles devoted to bodybuilding.

The testis manufactures testosterone using as a starting material the much-maligned cholesterol, which serves also as precursor for the body's life-supporting hormones of the adrenal gland. The main pathway for testosterone synthesis goes through the precursors DHEA, which has negligible androgenicity, and androstenediol, which is more androgenic. In another pathway, a weak androgen precursor, androstenedione, is converted to testosterone. The adrenal gland can also be a source of androgens and normally does produce a small amount in the course of making cortisonelike steroids and other hormones. There are pathological conditions in both men and women in which adrenal androgen production becomes overwhelming.

Enzymes present in the Leydig cells of the testis convert the cholesterol molecule to testosterone. Along the way, intermediates are produced that have androgenic activity. They have a local action in the testis, where they influence sperm formation, and they can be found, with testosterone, circulating in the blood enroute to other target cells around the body. DHEA is an intermediate widely publicized as having health-promoting benefits, including protection for the brain from senility and prevention of osteoporosis. Over the past 50 years, animal experiments have suggested that DHEA is a multipurpose hormone with antidiabetic, antiobesity, anticancer, immunoenhancing, memory-preserving, and antiaging effects. DHEA can be converted in the body to dehydroepiandrosterone sulfate (DHEAS), inactive as an androgen but also asserted to have myriad beneficial properties.

The DHEA/DHEAS complex is virtually inactive as an androgen. In the testis, conversion of DHEA to androstenediol enhances androgenicity substantially. In fact, androstenediol has about one and a half times the potency of testosterone. This means that some of the androgenic potency is lost during the conversion of androstenediol to testosterone. In another pathway, androgenicity is reduced when some of the androstenediol is converted into androstenedione. Then, some of the potency is restored in the final step, conversion of androstenedione to testosterone.

Sex hormone-binding globulin (SHBG) is a serum protein that, as its name implies, binds sex hormones. Because testosterone is not active in bound form, the more SHBG, the more testosterone is bound, and the less free testosterone is available to exert its androgenic activity. Given the importance of SHBG binding, the total testosterone value in the blood (bound plus free) is less significant for estimating bioactivity than the amount of free testosterone. Aging changes, therefore, are best followed by evaluating levels of SHBG. The presence of estradiol in men reduces the bioactive testosterone level because it raises the amount of SHBG. Hence, when a man's estrogen level is beginning to rise, his available testosterone will be reduced. An elevated level of estrogen is a common characteristic of octogenarians.

The factor that determines the potency of an androgenic molecule is its affinity for the androgen receptors of target cells. These receptors latch on to the free testosterone, or other androgen, in the circulating blood and transport the molecules to the cell nucleus where the steroid–receptor complex acts to change the pattern of protein synthesis. This converts nonstimulated cells to stimulated cells with a different pattern of cell growth and proliferation. Stronger androgens occupy more receptor sites and tend to displace weaker androgens.

Although androstenedione is a weak androgen, it fits into the scheme of things neatly because it can be converted to an estrogen (estrone), which in proper amounts has many important physiological functions in men. Testosterone can also be converted to the familiar estrogen estradiol. Estradiol plays a role in maintaining bone density, for example. When taken for bodybuilding or for other reasons, conversion of an androgen to excess estrogen can be a disadvantage because it can lead to feminizing side effects in men such as breast enlargement.

Androstenedione sprang to notoriety when it was found in baseball player Mark McGwire's locker during his record-breaking season of hitting 70 home runs. In this case, it was undoubtedly the convertibility of androstenedione to testosterone that had appeal, not its conversion to estrogen. The enzyme that carries out the conversion of androstenedione to estradiol is called aromatase because it adds an aromatic ring structure to the parent compound.

Some athletes are familiar with androstenediol, used for bodybuilding, believing it has the advantages of not converting directly to an estrogen and transforming more rapidly and more efficiently to testosterone. They are right. One study found that androstenediol could boost testosterone threefold compared to an equivalent amount of androstenedione. Both androgens enjoy the reputation of being safe to take because they are part of the normal process of testosterone synthesis within the body. That's probably acceptable reasoning as long as the resultant serum testosterone levels are kept within normal limits.

These precautions are not, however, a fully dependable safety net. After androgen is transformed to testosterone, the normal process brings about the conversion of testosterone to other androgen molecules by various tissues. The most important of these is the most potent androgen in the body, dihydrotestosterone (DHT). It is more than twice as potent as testosterone.

The conversion of testosterone to DHT requires the action of an enzyme known as 5α-reductase, which is found in several tissues including the prostate gland, other accessory sex organs, and the skin. This is a vital fact in considering HT for men because it is in the form of DHT that the body's androgens stimulate the prostate, perhaps the main cause for concern about men using testosterone. This is why it is important to avoid supraphysiological levels of testosterone that can result in exposure of the prostate to high DHT concentrations. Yet scientists have found that the application of a gel that delivers exogenous DHT to the body through the skin daily for three months does not stimulate the prostate gland in any measurable way, so there may be a wide safety range that protects the prostate or the observation period may be too short.

In the skin, DHT can cause overstimulation of the sebaceous glands, resulting in acne or of the hair follicles to cause hirsutism in women or accelerate male baldness patterns. Almost everyone, male or female, experiences some flare-up of acne or less severe skin eruptions when, at puberty, androgen production goes into high gear. This is not the result of testosterone directly, but of DHT. DHT is not only produced in these tissues by the action of 5α-reductase, but DHT accumulates in these tissues because they have androgen receptors with a strong affinity for the molecule.

The rate of DHT production is highest in the prostate and other accessory sex organs. The necessary enzyme for its production is present in the liver, but it does not accumulate there. Muscle does not have the 5α-reductase enzyme. Ultimately, testosterone is changed in the body to two principal active hormones: DHT, mostly in the male accessory sex organs, and estradiol, primarily in the liver, brain, and fat tissue.

The body has many circulating androgens that are part of the normal array of hormones, but each day a man produces mainly testosterone. For the principal androgens, the estimated production rates per day are: testosterone, 7 mg; androstenedione, 2.4 mg; and DHT, 0.3 mg. The sum of the actions of all these androgenic substances determines the overall biological impact of testosterone. This array of androgens does not mean that the body has a fail-safe system in case the testicular supply of testosterone falls. When testosterone production is interrupted, its precursor hormones and conversion products will disappear as well.

Finally, the body's androgens, testosterone, its precursors, and its conversion products, are metabolized to inactive forms, which are excreted in the urine or the feces in about equal proportions. They are cleared from the body rapidly after they are made so the production process in the testis must continuously maintain testosterone levels that are normal for each age group.

14 • Why should men consider androgen supplementation therapy?

It has not escaped men's attention that physical, mental, and emotional changes mark their advancing years. It may hit home when friends joke about their midlife crisis, senior moments, lack of concentration, tiredness, nervousness, or irritability. The idea that something can be done about these age-related symptoms is appealing and has sparked growing interest. Some men start to use androgens with great expectations, ranging from enhanced sexual prowess to youthful physical robustness. Elderly males hope that taking hormones will help them dodge the fate of old age: lethargy, memory loss, and frailty.

Hormone therapy is gaining popularity among men, but the benefits they anticipate from this therapy are sometimes unrealistic. The reality is that androgen replacement is no more of a pathway to eternal youth for men than HT is for menopausal women. Like any other medication, androgens carry benefits and risks and should be considered in this context.

As men age, their body composition changes. Lean body mass (mainly muscle) decreases while fat increases; muscle strength and energy levels also decline. There is no single cause for these changes. It is a delusion to think that such changes can be put off indefinitely by so simple a solution as testosterone supplementation. The search for the golden testicle has proven as futile as the quest for the fountain of youth.

Guinea pig testicle extracts and monkey glands are part of the early history of reproductive endocrinology, but modern science provides the facts that can correct misleading information and dispel false expectations. On one hand, one out of five older men maintains testosterone production in the normal range for healthy, virile young men; yet, they are still old. On the other hand, some normal young men with no symptoms of premature aging can have testosterone levels below the normal threshold. These observations reveal that there is more to youth and aging than hormone levels. This does not mean, however, that these levels are unimportant.

Many scientific studies support the conclusion that as men grow older, declining testosterone production can contribute to the characteristics of aging. The strongest evidence comes from the finding that testosterone treatment can reverse many age-related changes. Testosterone supplementation in older men can prevent the increase in body fat, arrest muscle loss, and actually increase lean body mass. This is due to testosterone's anabolic effect. This effect can be measured experimentally by the hormone's ability to stimulate muscle growth in laboratory animals and in men. Scientists are able to explain this muscle-building action on the basis of the ability of the hormone to stimulate muscle protein synthesis. Sophisticated methods of molecular biology have shown that, in the muscles of healthy young men, androgen supplementation improves the intracellular utilization of amino acids, the building blocks for proteins, and stimulates an increase in skeletal muscle protein synthesis. Although this has been measured in only a limited sample of bodily muscles, it can be assumed to apply throughout the body where skeletal muscles provide strength.

Heart muscle cells of both women and men also contain testosterone receptors. This would give these cardiac cells the ability to respond to androgens by accelerating the synthesis of proteins, but there are no clinical reports of testosterone supplementation leading to cardiac hypertrophy. In fact, laboratory findings suggest that dihydrotestosterone, not testosterone itself, may be responsible for stimulating protein synthesis in cardiac cells. Nevertheless, this possibility cannot be disregarded and is another reason that it is important to maintain testosterone supplementation within normal physiological limits.

Increase in skeletal muscle mass can be demonstrated when elderly men are treated with androgens. In one study, elderly, frail men received weekly testosterone injections, and the lean muscle mass in their legs increased by nearly 6% over 10 weeks. The muscle mass of men who had the hormone treatment and also exercised improved even more. Another study found the same beneficial effect on lean muscle mass and a decrease in body fat when testosterone was applied either as a gel or via a skin patch. In fact, delivering testosterone transdermally proved to be more effective than taking the weekly injections. The magnitude of the response depended on the dose. Men who used a testosterone gel that delivered 100 mg each day had a muscle mass increase of more than five pounds in 90 days, and when the dose taken was 50 mg per day, the muscle weight increase was half as large. The gel treatment resulted in loss of about two pounds of body fat over three months. The body composition benefits gained depend on the size of the dose and the resultant increase in serum testosterone level. This means that by accurately monitoring the testosterone level in the blood in response to treatment, it is possible to adjust the dosage to achieve maximal benefit from supplementation therapy.

For safety reasons, it is important that the testosterone concentration in the blood serum caused by the transdermal treatment remains in the normal range and does not rise to higher levels. Determining blood levels of testosterone is not a difficult laboratory procedure, but the doctor who orders the tests should know the most reliable methods of sampling and testing. Timing of blood sample collection is important, and the determination of both total testosterone and biologically active hormone provides valuable information to help decide whether treatment might be helpful and, if so, at what dose.

Increase in muscle mass does not automatically mean improvement in muscle strength, but studies have found increased strength is another benefit of testosterone treatment. Both upper and lower body muscle strength can be increased substantially in men using testosterone gel or patches. The increased strength can be achieved within 90 days in men using transdermal systems delivering either 100 mg or 50 mg/day. One relevant study continued the treatment for a full year and concluded that testosterone supplementation significantly improved upper body strength as measured by grip strength. This was evident after three months of treatment and continued throughout the year-long treatment period. Grip strength improvement is important because it is correlated with manual dexterity and how well older men can function in every-day life.

In addition to testosterone, other hormones have been tested for androgen replacement. These are usually analogues such as dihydrotestosterone, the conversion product that is several times more potent than testosterone. Dihydrotestosterone has the potential for stimulating the prostate (and possibly heart muscle cells), so it is not a good candidate for long-term use. However, it has the advantage of not being convertible in the body to estrogens. Thus the chances of breast enlargement that some men experience when using testosterone over a long period of time may be overcome by the use of dihydrotestosterone. Dihydrotestosterone may have a different effect in older men than testosterone, which the body does convert to estrogen. In short-term studies, dihydrotestosterone improved lower limb muscle strength, but this may be a case where the risks outweigh the gain.

Bone mineral density is another marker of aging influenced by testosterone. Peak bone mass is reached at an early adult age, and as men become older their bone density decreases. There are many reasons for this decrease including genetic factors, diet, exercise habits, and hormones. Excess alcohol consumption can contribute to bone loss. In the human body, the physiology of maintaining normal bone structure and bone mineral density is a dynamic process. At any age, there is a balance of bone formation and resorption. This is referred to as bone remodeling. The blood serum level of certain bone-specific enzymes can measure how remodeling is proceeding. With aging, this system can become imbalanced so that the cells that cause resorption outperform the cells that constantly replace bone. A person's bone status can be determined by a blood test to measure bone-specific enzymes, by a urinalysis to detect the by-products of bone remodeling, and by photometric measurements of bone density. Each of these tests is available in comprehensive health care facilities. Excess resorption can cause lower bone density, osteopenia, or even the more severe condition of osteoporosis. Osteoporosis in men leads to the risks of falls and fractures, a serious hazard of old age, even if the risk is lower than in postmenopausal women, who tend to lose a greater percentage of bone density with aging than men do.

Testosterone reduces bone resorption; this limits the loss of bone minerals and results in an increase in density. To determine whether there is bone mineral density deficiency to begin with and to measure the results of treatment, measurements are usually made of the lower spine vertebrae. According to most scientific reports, the bones of the hip are less likely to respond to testosterone treatment. Since, with aging, hip fractures are frequently the result of falls, this is a troubling limitation, but it may be overcome by designer androgens with greater affinity for the type of bone present in the hip.

Nevertheless, overall increase in bone density is a clear-cut benefit of testosterone supplementation. The greater the androgen deficiency to begin with, the greater the benefit that can be derived from supplementation therapy. The most significant improvement in bone mineral density occurs during the first year of therapy. Long-term treatment maintains bone mineral density at appropriate levels for a man's age.

Testosterone supplementation should not be considered a replacement for good dietary habits. As they become older, men need to maintain their intake of calcium and vitamin D. There are also nonhormonal bone-building drugs that can reverse low bone mineral density.

After age 40, men report having decreased sexual activity and less frequent intercourse. The decline continues into the 50s and beyond. There is also a loss of general interest in sex. Fifteen percent of men over 60 respond in questionnaires that they have no sexual interest; the corresponding rate in women of the same age is even higher.

Certainly testosterone is involved in the maintenance or loss of sexual desire or interest, but other medical and social factors are also responsible for these behavioral differences. This is true for both men and women. In stable marital relations, sexual activity depends on the attitudes and needs of two individuals. Sexual interest is also influenced by the general state of health and by other hormonal factors such as thyroid function or the hormones of the brain and pituitary gland. According to neurologists, a secondary effect of L-DOPA, which reaches the brain when used for the treatment of Parkinson's disease and other neurological disorders, is hallucinations including sexual fantasies and sometimes the general awakening of sexual interest.

Libido and sexual arousal are testosterone responsive. Testosterone administration to aging men can improve sexual activity by boosting libido. Within three months of androgen supplementation that restores testosterone levels to physiological values, the age-related decline in sexual interest and enjoyment can be reversed. Studies that have gone on for three years have demonstrated that this benefit can be maintained if the treatment is continued.

Erectile dysfunction (impotency) is more complicated than a simple androgen deficiency problem. The ability to have an erection is independent of testosterone levels. Fewer that 10% of men with erectile dysfunction have low testosterone. Moreover, increasing the baseline levels of older men with normal testosterone levels does not influence their erectile ability. Chronic conditions such as high blood pressure, arteriosclerosis (hardening of the arteries due to calcium deposition that reduces the blood vessel's flexibility), atherosclerosis (narrowing of the arteries due to lipid plaque formation on the vessel's inner wall), and diabetes contribute to the problem, and some of the drugs for the treatment of these conditions can also impair potency. Viagra or other drugs that help to cause and maintain blood flow to the vascular system of the penis are the treatment of choice. They work by permitting and maintaining engorgement of the penis. Before Viagra, mechanical devices were used to accomplish the same purpose.

Testosterone therapy results in increases in hematocrit and hemoglobin levels. As long as these values stay within normal limits, this activity is beneficial, particularly for men with low iron levels, even if they don't have frank anemia. Anemia in older men is a frequently unnoticed condition that can account for the chronic tiredness, mental apathy, and lethargy characteristic of many elderly people. These symptoms, however, should prompt a more complete endocrine work-up. Aging brings about a decline in other hormones as well as testosterone. Among these is thyroxin, the hormone of the thyroid gland. At any age hypothyroidism is characterized by a low energy level. Because of the overall pattern of aging changes in the endocrine system, some doctors prefer the term "partial endocrine deficiency" instead of "partial androgen deficiency" to describe the aging male. It is a more accurate characterization. PEDAM is the acronym for partial endocrine deficiency in aging men.

Sleep disorders are another symptom related to testosterone status that probably involves other endocrine factors as well. Thyroid and adrenal functions are certainly contributory, and melatonin, a brain hormone, is marketed as a sleeping aid. Melatonin levels are highest in infancy and then decline. What an intriguing prospect to be able to sleep like a baby! The improvement of sleep quality in elderly people by controlled release of melatonin has been claimed.

Most evidence concerning the beneficial effect of testosterone supplementation on sleep comes from responses of users. In survey studies, testosterone users report that their sleeping patterns improve when they are on therapy. Studies of interruption of breathing during sleep (sleep apnea), which causes sudden awakening have shown an increase in nightly episodes of sleep apnea in men taking testosterone supplementation. This may be an indication of a breathing disorder, and men using androgen therapy should be monitored for altered snoring habits.

The benefits of testosterone supplemention are not inconsequential. Maintaining muscle mass and strength and preventing the heart-stressing factor of abdominal fat deposition are good reasons for aging men to consider add-back therapy. In addition, the substantial evidence of other benefits, including bone mineral conservation and maintenance of blood iron stores, encourage the treatment of androgen deficiency. Behavioral changes concerning sexuality are more difficult to quantify. When treatment regimens keep serum testosterone levels within the physiologically normal range, for most men with androgen deficiency the benefits outweigh the risks.

15 • What are the AST choices for men?

Hormone replacement therapy for the aging man has a rich vocabulary. Some terms have been invented to fit specific products, and others are meant to convey a particular point of view about aging in men. Terms have even been adopted from the vernacular of the body-building cult, to whom the anabolic merits of testosterone are not unfamiliar.

The term "male menopause" is probably the easiest understood by the general public, even though it is derived from the words meaning the "end of menstruation." If mentioning andropause causes a puzzled gaze, adding, "male menopause" serves to clarify quickly. The old-fashioned term "male climacteric," also adopted from its female counterpart, still survives. Specialists in the field of andrology (the male equivalent of gynecology) have favored "andropause." Yet, it is still more likely to be found in crossword puzzles than in Florida cocktail party conversation. Conveying greater precision, "androgen deficiency in the aging male" (ADAM), or "partial androgen deficiency in the aging male" (PADAM) have evolved in professional usage. Even more precise is the term "partial endocrine deficiency in the aging male" (PEDAM). Although it is not often used, this term conveys the most complete information. It differs from the others because it encompasses endocrine changes other than androgens, such as the drop in thyroid hormone production, growth hormone, or insulin fluctuations with aging.

Hormone replacement therapy for men also has many names. Companies that market testosterone for hormone replacement prefer the term

TST (testosterone supplementation therapy) instead of HRT. Other ac-ronyms that have been used are AST (androgen supplementation therapy) and ART (androgen replacement therapy), not to be confused with the ART short for assisted reproduction technologies used in infertility treat-ment. You will hear about androgens, designer androgens, or selective androgen receptor modulators, and the abbreviated term "andro" (refer-ring to either androstenedione or androstenediol) has come into general usage. Steroids are referred to as "'roids" in the weight-lifting room.

Many of the substances and hormones involved in male HRT have long, complicated chemical names, so the use of acronyms (DHEA in-stead of dehydroepiandrosterone) or abbreviations ("dihydro" instead of dihydrotestosterone) is not uncommon.

The first attempts to use testosterone clinically were not successful and contributed to a bruised reputation for the therapy and reluctance on the part of many andrologists, gerontologists, and clinical endocrinologists to prescribe its use. Because testosterone is metabolized rapidly in the body, it proved to be ineffective when given orally or by injection. This is what led to the injectable pellet form of delivery. Under-skin pellets re-main available today containing 25 mg of a timed-release testosterone delivered over 4 months. With little information available concerning its pharmacodynamics, safety, and effectiveness, however, use of the pellet method has never gained popularity among prescribing physicians.

Two other forms of therapy were introduced when chemists were able to make certain modifications to the testosterone molecule that main-tained its androgenic properties but changed other characteristics. Oral activity was made possible by the synthesis of 17-alkylated derivatives, but this was an unfortunate chapter in testosterone supplementation history because these compounds caused liver damage, and this reputa-tion has lived on. Longer-acting injectable preparations were made possible by using a chemically modified testosterone with side chains attached to the basic molecule. This modification extends the duration of action within the body. These testosterone esters are still used today after first appearing in the 1950s.

By 2000, 20 injectable products containing testosterone or one of its longer-acting esters were available in the United States. Two of these, Depo-Testosterone and Delatestryl, accounted for 90% of the prescriptions filled for androgen injections. In 2000, total sales of injectable androgens were less than $22 million. Delatestryl and Depo-Testosterone combined captured $20 million of this small market. The active ingredient of Depo-Testosterone is the ester testosterone cypionate, and Delatestryl contains testosterone enanthate. The doses range between 200 and 400 mg taken biweekly or monthly. This schedule is a considerable improvement over earlier injectables that used a smaller ester, testosterone propionate and required an intramuscular injection two or three times a week.

Soon after injection, the body's enzymes remove the side chain from these esters and testosterone becomes available in the general circulation. In order for the testosterone concentration to stay above the threshold required for activity until the next injection, the initial level must be well above the normal range. These supraphysiological concentrations, the wide fluctuations in testosterone levels, plus the painful, repeated injections are major drawbacks for this means of drug delivery. Nevertheless, injectable testosterone esters have been on the market for many decades, mainly for the treatment of underdeveloped testes (hypogonadism) in boys or young men. Although prescription survey information can now distinguish between prescriptions written for this clear-cut indication and those intended to supplement testosterone in older men with partial androgen deficiency, this has not always been possible, so the historical use of testosterone by aging men is hard to measure.

In 2001 the sale of all testosterone prescription products in the United States reached $200 million, and the nonprescription purchase of prehormones which are converted by the body to testosterone has skyrocketed. Sold as nutritional supplements, these products (mainly DHEA and androstenedione) can hardly be kept in stock by the specialized stores that have sprouted up across the country selling vitamins and nonprescription pharmaceuticals.

When a transdermal testosterone gel (AndroGel) was marketed for the first time in the United States in 2000, even the company's president was surprised as the transdermal gel quickly took over the lion's share of the testosterone supplementation market. Within the first year after being introduced, it became a $100 million-a-year product, and its use is still growing rapidly. Known in the United States as AndroGel 1%, the clear, colorless, quick-drying gel contains 1% testosterone. It is applied on the skin of the upper arm, shoulders, or abdomen in quantities that contain 50 mg, 75 mg, or 100 mg of testosterone. The skin serves as a reservoir for the sustained release of testosterone into the general circulation beginning within 30 minutes. Single daily applications from packets with measured quantities can establish a steady state within a day or two and maintain testosterone blood levels in the normal range for many months. A drawback is the possibility of skin-to-skin transfer.

The FDA-approved labeling for AndroGel includes the statement that it can be used for replacement therapy in males for conditions associated with a deficiency or absence of endogenous testosterone. This clearly opens the door for use in hormone supplementation therapy in aging men. The widespread acceptance of the new gel product has boosted interest in male hormone treatment more generally, and several new topical gels are in development that use testosterone or other androgens.

Transdermal delivery is also the basis for skin patch products that release testosterone. There are two types of testosterone skin patches. One type is applied to the skin of the scrotum (Testoderm or Testoderm with Adhesives) to enhance the local concentration and simulate the natural site of production. The other type (Androderm or Testoderm TTS) is applied almost anywhere else on the body. Androderm is sold in patches containing 2.5 mg testosterone and, according to the dose prescribed, one, two, or three patches are applied every day. Testoderm TTS comes in 5-mg patches and is also changed every day. To mimic the normal diurnal rhythm of testosterone production, the patch is supposed to be applied in the early morning. The high-maintenance nature of this procedure does not help develop product loyalty, so it is not surprising that these patches quickly lost popularity to the gel as soon as the gel was introduced. Within one year, the volume of sales of all four of these established patch products combined reached no more than one-third that of AndroGel.

Androgenic prescription drugs taken orally are available for all hypogonadal indications, but their use is minimal and they are used only rarely for androgen replacement in aging men. Although 12 testosteronelike prescription products for oral use are sold in the United States, three dominate the market: Android-10, Halotestin, and the generic steroid fluoxymesterone. Android-10 is methyl testosterone prepared in 10-mg pills. The usual dose is 10–50 mg a day. Fluoxymesterone is contained in two products (Android F and Halotestin). Its name comes from the fact that a fluorine molecule is inserted into the basic testosteronelike structure. As fluorine belongs to the halogen group of chemicals, fluoxymesterone is sometimes referred to as a halogen-substituted steroid or halogenated steroid. Fluoxymesterone is very short acting (less than 10 hours) so pills need to be taken frequently during the day to maintain an effective blood level.

The Organon Company of Holland and its licensees in 90 countries market an oral androgen called Andriol. It is available in Canada but not in the United States. Andriol is an ester of testosterone with a lengthy side-chain (undecanoic acid). Because of this modification, it is absorbed differently from other oral medications. Instead of passing from the gastrointestinal tract to the liver, Andriol is absorbed from the gut into the lymphatic system. This results in bypassing the liver on first pass, thus avoiding hepatic toxicity. In the lymphatic system, the side chain is removed and the compound now becomes testosterone. It moves from the lymphatic system to the general blood circulation and interacts with target cell androgen receptors. Andriol (40-mg pills) is marketed for its anabolic properties in some countries and for partial androgen deficiency in aging men, in others. Because the testosterone ester is metabolized and cleared from the body quickly, the pills must be taken frequently during the day (total dose of 120–160 mg). Serum levels fluctuate widely. Andriol has been on the world market since 1978, but its introduction into the United States is unlikely. The anticipated market is too small to warrant the investment necessary to carry the drug through the required steps for FDA approval. Moreover, the enthusiastic claims of benefits found in advertisements for Andriol in some countries would not be allowed by the FDA without substantiating data.

Androgens available only through a doctor's prescription are FDA-approved for many characteristics including purity and batch consistency. They also have to meet strict regulations concerning proof of safety and efficacy before being put on the market. Even the packaging and its labeling are scrutinized for accuracy by the FDA before approval is granted. Unwarranted claims in advertising can result in withdrawal of approval. The most frequently used FDA-approved prescription androgens in the United States are listed in table 15.1.

In addition to androgens prescribed as FDA-approved drugs, a plethora of products are distributed in the United States as unregulated dietary supplements or are illegally imported and sold through the internet or other sources. These include products similar to those listed in table 15.1. Many are counterfeits of FDA-approved products. These are medicines that are deliberately and fraudulently mislabeled and can be totally useless or even harmful. The illegal market of steroids in the United States is believed to be $300–$400 million, virtually double that of the prescription drug market. Since steroids are classified as class 3 controlled substances under the Anabolic Steroid Control Act of 1990, acquiring an unauthorized steroid illegally not only puts you at a health risk but is also a felony. Ethical pharmaceutical companies maintain a wide array of products that can be safely used for androgen supplementation for aging men, and more are in the research pipeline. We are fortunate in the United States to have a drug distribution system that is structured, organized, and

Table 15.1. Prescription Androgens Used in the United States

Administration	Product name	Androgen used
Transdermal		
	AndroGel 1%	Testosterone
	Androderm	Testosterone
	Testoderm TTS	Testosterone
	Testoderm	Testosterone
	Testoderm/Adhesive	Testosterone
Injectable		
	Depo-Testosterone	Testosterone cypionate
	Delatestryl	Testosterone enanthate
Oral		
	Testred	Methyl testosterone
	Android 10	Methyl testosterone
	Halotestin	Fluoxymesterone
Subdermal		
	Pellets	Testosterone

Products with annual sales that exceed $1 million are listed.

regulated. It is a foolish decision to take the risks of using unproven and untested products for which unsubstantiated claims are made or to acquire them from countries with weakly regulated pharmaceutical markets.

Several scientific journal articles describe the use of human growth hormone (hGH) to offset the symptoms of partial endocrine deficiency in aging men. Growth hormone is a large, complex protein hormone produced by the pituitary gland. The hormone plays an important role in stimulating growth in children, and its prescribed use for this purpose in children with growth hormone deficiency is FDA approved. Because there is a gradual decline in growth hormone production with aging, some doctors have explored the benefits of replacing growth hormone in aging men. Improvements in just about every bodily function have been claimed, including reversal of the graying of hair, disappearance of wrinkles, and the prospect of a vigorous life beyond age 100.

We do not have personal experience with this suggested form of hormone therapy either in clinical practice or through research on growth hormone, so we leave it to others to discuss it in the books and articles written on the subject. Some writers are unabashed enthusiasts; others are severe critics. Replacement therapy in aging men (or women) is not an FDA-approved use of growth hormone. The effects of growth hormone treatment in adults with growth hormone deficiency described in the

FDA-approved package insert are limited to beneficial changes in body composition after treatment by daily self-injections for six months. Using growth hormone for a year could cost about $20,000, apart from the cost of careful medical management that is required. Medical follow-up on a regular basis should not be overlooked because of the possibility of potentially serious side effects. According to the manufacturers, experience with prolonged growth hormone treatment in adults is limited.

16 • The first designer androgen for men

"Designer estrogen" has become a household term. Now, the first designer androgen is in the research pipeline and may soon be available for use in androgen supplementation therapy.

The term "designer" applied to either an estrogen or an androgen is meant to convey the idea that the hormone is designed to maximize certain effects and minimize others. A designer estrogen or androgen is an engineered drug that possesses some, but not all, of the actions of the original hormone. Designer estrogens are also referred to as SERMs, which stands for "selective estrogen receptor modulators." This terminology is based on their mechanism of action at target cells.

A comparable term for a designer androgen would be a SARM, a selective androgen receptor modifier. They, too, appear to have an important future for replacement therapy. In this case the user population will be aging men. What the acronym SARM conveys is that the compound is able to select androgen receptors in some tissues and exert an androgenic or anabolic effect, while avoiding cell stimulation and proliferation at other locations.

Early work based on this principle led to development of antiandrogens that interfere with the action of testosterone without imparting replacement androgenic activity themselves. Cyproterone acetate is an antiandrogen that competes with testosterone at the receptor sites of target cells that are programmed to respond to androgens. Because of a lack of specificity (it can also modify other hormone receptors), cyproterone has limitations for clinical use. Proscar (finasteride) is another example of an androgen with greater selectivity. Prescribed for the treatment of prostate enlargement, finasteride lowers the level of dihydrotestosterone (DHT) in the prostate by inhibiting the action of the 5α-reductase enzyme. This is the enzyme that converts testosterone to dihydrotestosterone, the potent prostate-stimulating androgen. Because finasteride is not, itself, androgenic, this results in a tempering of the androgenic stimulation that promotes prostatic hypertrophy. It acts similarly on the androgen receptors of the hair follicles in the skin. With lower levels of DHT present, male-pattern hair loss can be delayed. This unexpected finding delighted the manufacturers of Proscar, and led to the introduction of another finasteride product, Propecia, sold specifically to combat male baldness.

Suppose you wanted to create a designer androgen for supplementation therapy for aging men. You could call together a group of experts, start with a strategy session, and ask, What would be the best goal in trying to engineer a designer androgen for androgen supplementation therapy? A wise conclusion would be to avoid the risk of prostate stimulation while maintaining the benefits of androgen replacement therapy. It is, after all, the fear of prostate hypertrophy and even prostate cancer that is the main restraint on greater use of androgens in aging. Your planning session might pursue the following logic: We know that androgenic stimulation of the prostate is the result of the conversion of testosterone to DHT, the much more powerful androgen. We also know that this transformation is brought about by the enzyme 5α-reductase, which is present in high concentration in prostate tissue. Let's design an androgen molecule that will be protected from the reductase enzyme but will still attach to the androgen receptors of other target cells. We would like a compound that retains its muscle-building and bone-strengthening activity, as well. In other words, we want an anabolic agent with selective androgenic activity, excluding the prostate.

This is exactly what scientists at the Population Council in New York, led by the late Carl Monder, a chemist, and endocrinologist Wayne Bardin, accomplished. The compound they settled upon and developed, sitting unused on the shelf of the Upjohn Company in Kalamazoo, Michigan, was 7α-methyl-19 nortestosterone, now better known by its acronym and trade name, MENT. Monder made the key discovery that the presence of the 7α-methyl group on the testosterone molecule prevents the 5α-reductase enzyme from transforming the molecule to DHT, or a similar derivative.

Joined by other Population Council scientists, particularly Kalyan Sundaram, Monder and Bardin did exhaustive studies on the chemistry, pharmacology, safety, and activity of the compound. In October 2000, the Population Council and Schering AG of Berlin announced a licensing agreement under which Schering would take over the development, manufacture, and worldwide marketing of MENT for hormone replacement therapy. The product is now being developed by Schering and has reached the stage of wide-scale clinical trials (phase III) to evaluate its effectiveness. Safety studies have already been completed satisfactorily. Barring unforeseen problems, MENT could be introduced for use in Europe by 2004, and in the United States a year later.

Like testosterone, MENT is not very active orally, so a different delivery system is required. The most advanced work has been with subdermal implants, similar to those used in NORPLANT contraceptive implants for women. This closes the circle that began many years earlier when Population Council scientists realized that long-term steroid hormone therapy can be delivered by using subdermal implants. When the research leading to NORPLANT began, we believed it could become an implant method of contraception that men could use. Several compounds were tested but none had sufficient potency or other characteristics required for an acceptable male implant method. The rate of release of testosterone, for example, was so rapid that an implant would empty too quickly to be practical. At the same time, new compounds were emerging for female contraception. The power of facts and data, therefore, prompted further development of an implant delivery system for a long-acting contraceptive method for women. More work on a comparable male method had to await further advances in the understanding of androgens and their mechanism of action. This has now been accomplished.

MENT has all the properties necessary for the subdermal implant method of delivery. It is a very potent androgen (10 times more potent than testosterone), and it is available in a form that remains stable when stored as a crystalline powder within the capsule at body temperature. It is soluble in the plastic matrix that makes up the capsule wall. This means that it will be released from the capsule at a steady rate depending on the differential between its solubility in the matrix and the surrounding bodily fluids. As a subdermal delivery system, it reaches the general circulation avoiding a first pass to the liver, which could cause rapid inactivation or liver toxicity. The high potency means that a capsule of practical dimensions can hold a quantity of the hormone powder that will last a long time. By modifications of the capsule matrix, the rate of release can be controlled to make implants that are long-acting in order to provide long-term effectiveness. The effective life of MENT implants is at least six months. Consequently, two semiannual visits to a doctor's office for capsule placement could replace daily pill or gel use, weekly patch application, or monthly injections of testosterone products. By this method, a man can obtain a full year of low-maintenance, uninterrupted hormone replacement therapy. The six-month intervals also provide good timing for check-ups that men should schedule anyway while on androgen replacement therapy. The capsule dimensions are small enough to permit placement under the skin through a narrow trochar, using local anesthetic applied to the insertion site, usually the upper arm. The entire procedure takes less than three minutes. Properly done, the removal of empty capsules is equally simple. MENT is also being studied for use in gel or patch delivery systems to provide choices in therapy methods.

Detailed information on the advantages of MENT for partial androgen deficiency in aging men must await the completion of more clinical trials. Meanwhile, studies have been done on some key issues. Like testosterone, MENT is a potent suppressor of pituitary gonadotrophin secretion so that it can suppress testicular hormone production as well as sperm production (its potential as a male contraceptive is not being overlooked). The compound serves as an excellent add-back therapy because it is 10 times more active than testosterone. In contrast to testosterone, its action is prostate sparing. It retains the testosteronelike characteristic of being convertible to an estrogen (7α-methyl estradiol), so that it can prevent bone loss, osteopenia, and osteoporosis. Although specific studies have not yet been carried out to measure the effects of MENT on body composition, muscle strength, or sexual interest and behavior, there is no reason to believe that it behaves differently from testosterone or other androgens in these respects. Indeed, its high potency may provide extra strength to elicit these favorable responses. Clues that this may be expected come from animal studies in which MENT is five times more potent than testosterone in maintaining sexual behavior. Because of this high potency, only a low daily dose of MENT is needed, making feasible delivery by an implant system.

To assure stability during storage, implants are filled with a chemically pure powder of the acetate form of 7α-methyl-19 nortestosterone, but as it is released from the implant into circulation, the acetate part of the molecule is rapidly lost. The compound is immediately converted to MENT itself as soon as it enters the body.

The effects of long-term use of MENT by men is not known, but animal studies are reassuring concerning long-term safety. MENT does not bind to the carrier protein, sex hormone binding globulin (SHBG), which enhances the solubility of other steroid sex hormones in the blood serum. This assures its bioavailability and fast clearance from the body. As MENT is cleared rapidly in humans, no accumulation would be expected.

The single implant or two implants that will most likely be the preferred dose used for androgen supplementation will release 0.5–0.7 mg of MENT per day. Considering that the estimated testicular production rate of testosterone by normal young men is 7 mg per day and that MENT is about ten times as potent as testosterone, this will provide almost complete androgen add-back for the aging male at a very constant rate, without the need for strict compliance or adherence to a precise dosing schedule. Achieving this with the knowledge that receptors in the prostate, skin, and hair follicles will not amplify the androgenicity of this designer androgen will be a major advance for male HRT and will undoubtedly trigger the search for compounds with similar advantages. Implants and other delivery forms of MENT will have several uses in andrology, including the treatment of hypogonadism, male contraception, therapy for delayed puberty in boys, as well as for replacement therapy for partial androgen depletion in aging men.

17 • Can men safely use AST?

An accurate term to describe the hormonal changes of older men is "partial androgen deficiency." Androgens stimulate male anatomical structures such as the prostate gland and also effect other masculine characteristics. These hormones also influence many general metabolic functions, including bone mineral density, maintenance of muscle cells, and the hemoglobin content of blood. Strictly speaking, androgens cannot be called "male hormones" because the ovaries and adrenal glands of women also produce them.

There are several androgenic hormones produced by the body or that chemists can synthesize in the test tube, but the obvious androgen to use for male replacement therapy is testosterone, the principal hormone produced by the testis. The level of testosterone production decreases in men as they age. By the time a man reaches 70 years of age, his level of biologically active testosterone has fallen to half its level at age 20. Whether this is the defining cause of aging changes, however, remains controversial. Although studies of large numbers of men show that in the general population, free testosterone (the component of the circulating hormone that is biologically active) concentrations decline by up to 1% per year, some doctors believe that a falling testosterone level is a measure of ill health in aging men. This point of view suggests that the percentage of healthy older men who need testosterone therapy is low. Alternatively, it is argued that all men that have testosterone values in the low or below normal range could benefit from add-back therapy. The mounting evidence published in some of the most respected scientific journals supports this position.

Use of androgen supplementation is increasing. Partly, this growing interest is because of the changing demographics of America. Baby boomers are now over 50. During the next 25 years the elderly population (age 65 and over) will increase by more than 50%, according to the U.S. Census Bureau. Market analysts believe that approximately 5 million American men, mainly in the older age groups, have lower than normal levels of testosterone. By 2025, the total could be 15 million.

In 2001 the sale of testosterone prescription products in the United States was twice as high as the previous year's total. When a transdermal testosterone gel (AndroGel) was marketed for the first time in the United States, it immediately gained widespread acceptance for testosterone supplementation in older men with partial androgen deficiency.

Although hormone replacement for men is gaining popularity, the question of its safety often arises. Are there risks that would outweigh potential benefits? The Controlled Substances Act of the United States classifies testosterone and similar anabolic agents as schedule III controlled substances. This classification means that while the substance has a useful and legitimate medical purpose, it should not be used without proper medical supervision, and the Drug Enforcement Administration has the authority to control its distribution. The Anabolic Steroid Control Act of 1990 criminalizes sale and possession of any anabolic steroid intended for nonmedical use.

There are three main reasons for these constraints and for the reluctance of some doctors to give testosterone supplementation to men: potential for liver damage, fear of prostate stimulation, and concern about its effect on the heart. Even today, many doctors, especially urologists, hold these concerns. The stimulatory action of testosterone on the prostate gland is so well known that urologists concerned with prostate cancer or benign prostatic hypertrophy (BPH) would be likely, for this reason alone, to veto a patient's decision to consider the use of testosterone supplemental therapy. This is understandable considering that for a long time the only treatment for prostate cancer began with orchiectomy (surgical removal of the testes) in order to eliminate the body's source of testosterone. The discovery of a hormonal treatment for prostate cancer that suppresses testicular production of testosterone earned for the late Charles Huggins of the University of Chicago the only Nobel Prize in Medicine ever awarded to a urologist. This recognition, in 1966, awarded for the discovery of a method to eliminate the body's testosterone, was an ironic twist considering that 27 years earlier the Nobel had gone to two German chemists for discovering how to synthesize testosterone in the laboratory.

A more sophisticated treatment, essentially chemical castration, is achieved by the administration of an analogue of a brain hormone (another Nobel Prize-winning discovery) that eliminates the function of the testis as efficiently as the surgeon's scalpel. Nowadays, castration is not a first-line treatment so that men who have been diagnosed with prostate cancer may undergo surgical removal of the cancerous prostate gland, various types of radiation therapy, or watchful waiting with no treatment at all. This is the choice triad given to patients; with each the body's own testosterone-producing system (the gonads) remains intact.

If physicians do not believe it is necessary to remove the endogenous testosterone source from men with prostate cancer, why would it be a hazard with respect to prostate stimulation to keep the hormone's level within physiological range in normal men with partial androgen deficiency? This reasoning has led to a greater willingness to accept the idea that men can be given testosterone, as long as the circulating level stays within normal limits. In adult men, this is between 3 ng/ml and 8 ng/ml of blood. Keeping within this range is feasible with products now marketed, regardless of age or body weight. Studies with AndroGel, for example, found that over a six-month period, 9 out of 10 men maintained serum testosterone levels within the normal range. Transdermal patches such as Androderm and Testoderm can also deliver testosterone in this controlled fashion. Moreover, we now have the prospect of the first designer androgens (see chapter 16) that suppress and replace the body's own testosterone and have all the beneficial androgenic and anabolic effects but do not stimulate the prostate.

Cardiologists have generally believed testosterone to be a heart-unfriendly hormone. Because coronary artery disease is seen more frequently in men than in women, it was thought that testosterone may play a causal role in this increased risk. Now, it appears the opposite may be true. Research has shown that testosterone reduces the incidence of several factors associated with heart disease. Testosterone treatment decreases total cholesterol levels significantly and improves the ratio of high-density lipoprotein (HDL) to low-density lipoprotein (LDL) cholesterol. Men in the general population with higher testosterone levels have higher levels of HDL cholesterol and lower levels of triglycerides, another heart-risk component of the blood's lipid profile. Moreover, there are other blood lipid factors that carry risk for coronary artery disease, and their level is also reduced by testosterone.

There is gathering evidence of other heart-sparing actions of testosterone. In otherwise healthy men, lower than normal testosterone levels over time can lead to accumulation of abdominal fat, a factor generally believed to increase the risk for atherosclerosis. This can be prevented or reversed by the administration of testosterone. Several studies have found that testosterone reduces exercise-induced ischemia (oxygen deprivation) in the heart muscle of men with established coronary artery disease. This beneficial result is due to the direct effect of testosterone on vasodilation; it improves relaxation of coronary arteries, which is beneficial but is impaired in coronary heart disease. Low doses of testosterone may relieve chronic angina, the pain that signals heart disease and can be incapacitating. In research on this subject, men with angina taking an exercise stress test showed a significant increase in exercise time when taking testosterone compared to when they did not take a testosterone supplement.

Cardiovascular disease is a major cause of illness and death in older men. Before there will be general acceptance of testosterone therapy, the safety of androgen replacement for heart disease factors needs to be firmly established, including an analysis of long-term effects. Much has been published on this subject, and more research is in progress. Until now, the available data give reassurance that from the cardiovascular perspective, testosterone is safe for older men experiencing partial androgen deficiency.

Androgens carry a bad reputation concerning liver toxicity. This comes from the past history of testosteronelike medications. A particular type of synthetic androgen, referred to as 17α-alkylated androgens (for example, methyl testosterone), became popular for treatment of hypogonadism. Their popularity was generated by the convenience of oral effectiveness, a welcomed alternative to frequent, sometimes painful injections or the insertion of pellets under the skin, a form of delivery that proved to be erratic and inconsistent. The orally effective alkylated androgens pass directly from the gastrointestinal tract to the liver. This creates a high initial bolus of the drug reaching the liver, without the benefit of first having the dilution effect of passing into the general circulation. With long-term use, these alkylated compounds taken orally can cause an increase in certain liver enzymes, jaundice, and liver damage. They have even been implicated in liver cancer. There is one testosterone ester (Andriol) used as oral medication that avoids the bolus impact on the liver because it is absorbed through the body's lymphatic system. Although it is orally active, it is not very potent and requires multiple doses a day. It is marketed in Canada, Europe, and Asia but not in the United States.

In 2001 six oral androgen products that use 17α-alkylated compounds were still marketed in the United States but are rarely used. The total volume of their sales was less that 2% of the total prescription sale of androgens in the United States. They have disappeared from use in Europe. The experience with the alkylated derivatives of testosterone is the reason that some doctors believe that testosterone may interfere with liver function. Hence, the reputation concerning liver toxicity lives on. The androgen used in the transdermal products that constitute the bulk of androgen prescription sales do not produce these adverse effects. The modern testosterone products on the market were carefully evaluated before receiving FDA approval and have a clear record with respect to liver toxicity.

Testosterone is also known to stimulate the production of erythrocytes (red blood cells), thereby increasing the blood's oxygen-carrying capacity. Called hematopoiesis or erythropoiesis, this effect is one of the reasons for the illegal use of androgens by athletes. As stimulation of erythrocyte production continues, the percentage of blood volume occupied by the red bloods cells increases. This is measured as the hematocrit, and it can become a health risk for clot formation if it exceeds normal limits and the blood becomes overly viscous. With older injectable androgen products that increased testosterone levels above normal, this was a problem that required close regular monitoring of the hematocrit, but the newer transdermal delivery systems maintain more physiological levels of testosterone and produce less erythropoietic stimulation. Testosterone does not have a direct effect on normal clotting characteristics of blood but could affect the action of blood-thinning drugs like coumadin, a medication frequently used by elderly men, resulting in the need for dose adjustment.

As interest in testosterone supplementation in older men has increased, the attention given to the safety issues has grown significantly, and it has become evident that the pattern of side effects with the older, alkylated androgens does not apply to testosterone, particularly when used in a transdermal delivery system which avoids the first pass to the liver. The number of scientific studies of testosterone supplementation is impressive and makes it possible to draw evidence-based conclusions on issues that were previously uncertain. The weight of scientific evidence confirms that many of the older fears of testosterone therapy are unfounded. Doses of testosterone or other androgens that maintain an older man's bioavailable testosterone level within physiological range can be taken safely. The feasibility and convenience of safe androgen supplementation is enhanced by the availability of user-friendly, transdermal delivery systems. The prospect of designer androgens, of which MENT is the leading example, promises even greater confidence in the safety of hormone replacement therapy for men.

18 • Should aging men use nonprescription androgens?

Barry Bonds wiped out Mark McGwire's home run record just three years after it was set. *Muscle Builder* magazine would be thrilled to have either one of them on its cover. Spindle-legged and paunchy Babe Ruth reigned as Sultan of Swat for 34 years before lanky Roger Maris unseated him in 1961. The Maris record held for 37 years. When Bonds was heading toward his record 73 home runs, a baseball league official, concerned about the possible use of steroids by players to build greater muscle mass, is quoted as saying, "Look at these guys. Look at their arms, their upper bodies, their thighs. All of a sudden they're huge. You can't do that in the gym." After Bonds started the next season with four homers in the first two games, his team trainer said, "They all take vitamin supplements. Barry does that, uses protein drinks, over-the-counter stuff." By the end of the season the players union had agreed to random testing for steroids, and a noted sports orthopedist, James Andrews, was quoted as saying that the bulking up and the increased injuries in baseball are attributable to steroids and supplements.

Professional athletes don't like to talk about steroid use, so we are left to speculate. The quantity of nonprescription steroids purchased by professional and amateur athletes, including high school athletes, is mind boggling. One study put the annual dollar amount at $800 million. That's four times as much as the total spent on all prescription androgens combined.

The reason athletes take these products is to crank up their testosterone levels to enhance muscle building. They cannot use testosterone itself because that would be illegal; it is a prescription drug regulated by the FDA. The way around this ban is to turn to the easily available prehormones and let the body do the final conversion. Testosterone has well-known anabolic (protein build-up) effects in addition to its role of maintaining male characteristics. It does this through stimulation of muscle protein development by more efficient utilization of amino acids (the building blocks of proteins) in muscle cells. Androstenedione or DHEA (dehydroepiandrosterone), the two main prehormones used for muscle building, can be bought over the counter in any GNC store or a multitude of other outlets. Type in "andro" on the Internet and you will bring up links to 131,000 web sites. Most of them relate to androstenedione. There are products, suppliers, clubs, newsletters, or chat groups to choose from. Promotional material concentrates on how far and how fast androstenedione enhances testosterone. The most extreme promotional claim we could find spoke of a 400% boost above normal range. One promised 134% testosterone increase in thirty minutes.

The Mark McGwire disclosure in 1998 that he routinely used androstenedione prompted several studies on its effectiveness. Scientists evaluated the testosterone-enhancing and muscle-building effects of androstenedione or DHEA in doses from 100 to 300 mg a day, the range recommended by most products on the market. The results fell far short of expectations. Scientific studies at major universities find little or no difference between androstenedione and placebos. But if androstenedione doesn't work any better than sugar pills, where did those guys get those big muscles? Vitamins? Protein drinks? In the gym, as they claim? And how do you explain the former East German Olympic team whose doctor described the routine use of androstenedione by nasal spray in the years that the East German teams won most of the medals? Were they deluding themselves into record-setting performances?

While athletes are convinced that these drugs are effective, scientists cannot find supporting data. Eager to believe the promised benefits, many athletes accept anecdotal information that promises safety and spectacular results. Scientists, on the other hand, have not obtained data to support those claims. They expect to see, for example, meaningful differences in testosterone blood levels if someone uses androstenedione.

One study, sponsored by the Office of the Commissioner of Baseball and the Players Association, was done by Benjamin Leder and colleagues at Harvard University. Young men took either 100 mg or 300 mg doses of androstenedione daily. The lower dose had no effect. The higher dose did cause a transient rise (34%) in serum testosterone level, and then the level fell back down again as the estrogen level rose (testosterone is rapidly converted to estradiol). The increase did not come close to the exaggerated claims made for many androstenedione products. Another study done at Iowa State University, home of the perennial NCAA wrestling champions, found no increase at all with 300 mg daily doses, taken in divided doses of 100 mg three times a day. Other studies were carried out in Texas, Florida, California, and Tennessee, all at universities with strong programs in sports medicine (to say nothing of their football teams). Their conclusions were similar. The Texas authors reported that oral androstenedione did not increase plasma testosterone concentrations and had no anabolic effect on muscle protein metabolism. The Tennessee researchers studied physiological and hormonal influences of androstenedione and androstenediol supplementation in men 35–65 years old. They found that 12 weeks of androstenedione use did not differ from placebo with respect to body composition or muscular strength. Total testosterone levels increased 16% after 1 month of use, but by the end of 12 weeks they returned to pretreatment levels. There were no benefits noted in the androstenediol group. The Florida project concluded that neither DHEA nor androstenedione elicits a statistically significant increase in muscle mass, strength, or testosterone levels in healthy adult men over a 12-week period. The doses used in all these studies followed the manufacturer's recommended dose of 100–300 mg per day.

Either the country's scientists are designing their studies improperly, or the country's young athletes are downing hundreds of millions of dollars worth of useless pills that might even be harmful. We cannot discount the possibility that the design of the studies could be misguided or confounded in several ways. For example, the age of the men studied could be an important variable. This has been tested, however, and proves not to be an important factor. In one study that included men 30–56 years old, there were no age-related differences in response. Or, the initial testosterone status of subjects in the studies could influence the results. Generally, men with normal testis function were enrolled because the primary objective of these investigations was to determine if young athletes were deriving any benefits from the use of androstenedione. It could be misleading to generalize the results to include older men, particularly aging men with partial androgen deficiency.

Another issue is whether the products used were pure and whether the subjects complied with the intended schedule. In a UCLA study, the investigators learned that there was a contaminant in the androstenedione they had used. They subsequently tested nine different brands of androstenedione in 100-mg doses. They found wide variations in overall content; the androstenedione levels ranged from 0 to 103 mg. One product even contained some testosterone. This is not entirely surprising since these products are classified as "nutrients" and are therefore exempt from FDA scrutiny. Since the distributors do not claim their products treat, cure, or prevent a disease, they can slip though this loophole in the country's regulatory procedures. Consequently, purity, batch consistency, and claims of effectiveness are not supervised.

The answer to why scientific information and anecdotal information differ so widely may lie in the difference between how androstenedione products are actually used by athletes seeking a competitive edge and the recommended doses used in scientific investigations. Although the recommended dose is usually around 100 mg, it is apparently common practice for athletes or body builders to exceed this by far, sometimes taking 500 mg a day. In addition, the practice of "stacking" is commonplace. This refers to taking several anabolic agents at the same time, using the prehormone steroids and other ingredients believed to be testosterone boosters. Claims include that these substances, usually of plant origin, prevent the conversion of testosterone to estrogen, act as antiestrogens, or stimulate the body's own production of testosterone. This sort of dosing has never been tested scientifically. It is possible that when scientific trials were set up to conform with recommended doses, the tests carried out around the country were done with amounts of androstenedione far below what athletes are actually using.

With this possibility in mind, scientists have begun to do studies using large, suprapharmacological doses. According to initial reports, they do appear to show the changes athletes are looking for, or which could benefit the aging male. While this may be the answer to the huge disconnect between what scientists believe and what users of androstenedione believe, it reopens the question of safety. The smaller recommended doses have generally been accepted as being benign, but studies with even these low doses have raised some warning signals. One finding is that the level of high-density lipoprotein cholesterol decreases, a concern in the risk of atherosclerosis and heart disease. Estrogen levels increase, which can lead to breast enlargement and other problems. Another hormonal warning sign is the significant increase in DHT levels after only 4 weeks of taking 100 mg of androstenedione. DHT is the potent androgen created from testosterone by an enzyme found in the highest concentration in the prostate gland. The major target organ of DHT is the prostate, where it can stimulate growth and cause hypertrophy. Although the studies found no significant change in prostate function (measured by the prostate-specific antigen test) after one month, more prolonged supplementation could result in detectable changes in prostate function and size. The association between anabolic steroid use and long-term health risks in former athletes has been studied, and premature mortality has been found to be an outcome. The three issues of concern that may be causal factors for this unsettling finding are adverse effects on the cardiovascular system, mental health problems, and increased cancer risk. Apparently, while the recommended doses of androstenedione may be benign, at the doses actually being used androstenedione may not be innocuous.

The other popular prehormone, DHEA, and its sulfate ester DHEAS, have a scientific uncertainty of their own. When taken by young men for serum testosterone enhancement and body strengthening, these prehormones fail the test of scientific scrutiny. A study led by Gregory Brown at Iowa State University concluded that DHEA ingestion does not enhance serum testosterone concentrations. Other specific testosterone-dependent end-point studies have had negative results as well. DHEA does not maintain bone mineral density, for example, when used by older men over six months at doses targeted to restore circulatory levels to levels that are normal for younger men.

These findings do not mean, however, that DHEA can be written off so quickly. For decades, animal experiments have suggested that DHEA can serve many health-promoting functions that may not be related to its conversion to testosterone. There is evidence that it prevents age-related loss of the body's ability to fight of infections. Since it can be found in the brain, DHEA may influence processes of memory and cognition. Some studies have found evidence for anticancer and antiaging affects. Consequently, DHEA advocates include not only athletes interested in bulking up, but endocrinologists interested in understanding the process of aging. Their views are backed by animal studies and also by reports on the beneficial effects of DHEA or DHEAS when they are used to restore normal levels in men or women who have low levels. Study results, however, are not consistent.

The body's production of DHEA drops from about 30 mg a day at age 20 to less than 6 mg a day at age 80. Advocates of DHEA use are impressed by reports that mortality rates are inversely related to DHEA levels. In other words, old men with higher DHEA levels live longer and function better. Advocates believe that replacement therapy can yield the benefits derived from having a higher DHEA level. These are very attractive potential benefits for a drug that has no evident risks. Compared with placebo, DHEA has no effect on serum lipids, liver or kidney function, or other markers of toxicity. A study in France concluded that a daily dose of 25–50 mg DHEA is safe in elderly men. At most, a cautionary note may be that estrogens increase but remain within the normal range for men. So, in spite of the inconsistency and the fact that some studies show no definitive evidence for the benefits of providing DHEA to healthy men with age-related decline of DHEA production, its popularity lingers on. The nothing-to-lose philosophy seems to drive this acceptance, but the overall scientific basis is weak. An aging man who is inclined to initiate androgen replacement therapy is better advised to do so with the advice and monitoring of a doctor, rather than trying a do-it-yourself approach.

19 • Sex and the aging man

On the assumption that many readers may turn to this chapter first before deciding whether to read the book, we'll start with the encouraging news that androgen supplementation therapy (AST) can increase sexual interest and improve sexual function. It is also possible for men on androgen supplementation to retain adequate sperm production to remain fertile if they wish to. Alternatively, there are AST regimens that reduce sperm counts sufficiently to make fertility nearly impossible. In other words, AST may be able to double as a male contraceptive.

Male fertility does not necessarily decline with aging, in distinct contrast to female fertility. The term "partial androgen deficiency in the aging man" is coined specifically to exclude a decline of fertility with aging. The reason for this is that the hormone-producing capacity of the testis is not linked to sperm production, so even though hormone production may be declining, sperm production can continue.

The ovary functions very differently from the testis; hormone and egg production are linked through their anatomical association as different parts of the same structure, the ovarian follicle. Moreover, in addition to the decline in fertility as the follicle count decreases with age, there is also a loss of egg fertilizability. Genetically built into the biology of the ovary is an aging factor that affects the eggs directly. This does not happen to sperm. Even if there is a decline in total sperm count with aging, this change is not reflected in a decreased ability of the sperm of aging men to fertilize an egg. This has not been easy to prove because older men tend to reproduce with older women, and it is difficult to eliminate from studies of large populations the influence that the declining fertility of aging women has on a couple's reproductive ability.

The contrast of male gamete (sperm) performance is striking. In artificial insemination cycles, fertilization rates and embryo quality are the same regardless of the age of the male providing the semen sample. This does not mean that total sperm produced remains the same with aging. Several studies have found evidence of decreasing sperm count with advancing age, although this has not been a consistent finding. A decrease of about 2.5 million sperm per cc semen per year of age, on average, was reported in one publication (see table 19.1). A decline of this limited magnitude would not be likely to reduce a man's fertility. In fact, the very same study found that age did not affect the ability to fertilize. I was particularly interested in this finding because it helped explain an observation I made in rural India years earlier, when I counseled infertile couples. Many of the couples had been trying to conceive for years, unaided by professional guidance, so that their average age was rather advanced. My first impression was that many of the couples were simply too old, both husband and wife, to expect successful pregnancies. The men tended to be older than their wives, as is customary in rural India. In some cases the age difference was large. It has always puzzled me that the men, with only an occasional exception, had sperm counts, motility, and viability similar to what would be expected of younger men.

Since that time, considerable scientific attention has been given to the effect of aging on sperm counts. As already mentioned, some studies have found a decline in count with aging; others have not. Many factors influence sperm counts. An important factor to consider in interpreting a semen sample is the period of prior abstinence. Unless that is kept constant, it is misleading to compare sperm counts from one set of data to another. If the ejaculate-free interval before sample collection is kept constant, sperm counts comparisons can be considered valid. Table 19.1 is an example, taken from a well-designed study in California.

Most andrologists agree that aging men may have a decline in sperm count but that they retain their fertility, and their sperm do not lose fertilizing capacity. Taking some form of AST can have an influence on this situation. It will not influence the sperm's fertilizing capacity, but it could have an impact on sperm number. In addition to its other androgenic and anabolic functions, testosterone normally plays a role in sustaining sperm production. With adequate doses of the right combination of ste-

Table 19.1. Sperm Counts and Fertilization Rates of Men Providing Semen Samples for Artificial Insemination

	All men 22–64 years	Men over 50 years
Average age	41.6 years	54.6 years
Sperm count (per cc semen)	207 million	159 million
Fertilization rate	60%	58%

All men: 558 samples; over 50 years: 60 samples. Sperm count average of the older men is considered significantly lower than counts of the younger men. Fertilization rates are not significantly different. Data from Paulson R et al. (2001).

roid hormones, the production of pituitary gonad-stimulating hormones, the chemical messengers that regulate the testis, is shut down, so that testis production of both its own hormones and sperm cease. With time, however, the counts will rebound even though the steroid treatment is continued. The explanation is that if the testosterone level (from the external source) is high enough, this can act to maintain spermatogenesis independent of the pituitary's control.

Rebound should be considered when initiating testosterone supplementation. When testosterone levels are maintained within normal levels, there will be no negative effect on existing sperm-producing capacity. It may improve somewhat. At large doses of exogenous testosterone, spermatogenesis may be suppressed through feedback inhibition of the pituitary's testis-stimulating hormones (luteinizing hormone and follicle-stimulating hormone). It cannot be assumed that rebound will not take place. Consequently, depending on a man's sexual activity, if protecting against pregnancy is desired, contraception should always be considered when a man is on testosterone supplementation. With designer androgens now in the research pipeline, automatic contraception will be built in as a bonus of AST. MENT, the super-androgen that is likely to be the first of these designer androgens on the market, will stop sperm production and keep it suppressed during treatment. For a man who wants to maintain his fertility, this would not be a wise choice of supplementation therapy. A man in these circumstances who initiates any regimen of testosterone supplementation should include periodic screening of a semen sample as a part of his medical supervision.

Fertility may be less relevant for most aging men than interest in sexual activity and performance. Although measurements of these factors are less quantitative than sperm counts or testosterone values, there is uniformity in the findings of many studies by leading endocrinologists and other medical specialists around the world. Studies have found that testosterone therapy can cause a significant increase in sexual desire, increase in enjoyment of sex with the same partner, increase in number of erections per month, more satisfaction with the duration of erection, and increase in the frequency of ejaculations. These studies have all used questionnaires administered before treatment and at monthly intervals during treatment. Can we believe in the results of this type of information gathering? To be blunt: Should we be suspicious about macho bragging tendencies about sex? There may be an element of concern about this, but the results have been so consistent in study after study, that their basic validity should not be questioned. In fact, some studies have added information obtained from the sexual partners of men using AST, and this information is confirmatory. In addition, quantitative measurements have been added on nocturnal penile tumescence along with diaries and questionnaires. These results are also confirmatory. Spontaneous nocturnal erection is a physiological androgen-dependent phenomenon. Both testosterone and MENT can stimulate significant increases in this measure of sexual interest and activity.

The package insert for AndroGel, now the most widely used testosterone supplementation product on the market, includes an FDA-approved claim that three months of treatment produces significant improvement in libido (measured by sexual motivation, sexual activity, and enjoyment of sexual activity). It also states that penile erection increased as did satisfaction with the duration of erection, according to subjective information provided by the users. This is not the same as a claim that AndroGel can be used to treat erectile dysfunction, but there is substantial evidence that it can enhance participation in sexual activities.

Erectile dysfunction in older men is rarely caused by testosterone deficiency, so sexual performance related to this condition (impotency) will not be improved by supplementation therapy. Viagra is not a hormone treatment. It works through a totally different mechanism involving an effect on the small blood vessels of the penis.

In older men, improvement of libido often is accompanied by improvement in psychological well-being and mood. Psychologists specializing in sexual behavior have developed comprehensive testing methods, used in clinical practice to evaluate patients and their progress. Findings from clinical practice confirms the findings of endocrinologists and andrologists concerning the behavioral effects of testosterone supplementation. In older men, the decrease in testosterone with age is closely correlated with a decline in sexual enthusiasm or libido. This is measured in terms of decrease in frequency of sexual thoughts, frequency of desire for sex, easiness to become aroused, degree of coital erections, and frequency of nocturnal erections. Mood changes tending toward depression and loss of interest in many activities have also been monitored. These behavioral characteristics are measurably improved with supplementation therapy. In one study, outcomes were examined among men with low testosterone who received supplementation therapy and others who declined the treatment. After two years, 80% of those receiving testosterone had increased libido, and the majority of those who did not accept treatment had a decline in libido.

For almost a century, since hormones were discovered, there have been attempts to promote the idea of rejuvenation through the use of hormones. In fact, early endocrinologists were fascinated with the idea of transferring the potency of animal testes to aging men. The testis was viewed as the repository of youth, and quackery abounded. Today data derived from well-designed clinical studies are available to substantiate claims and define the limits of expectation. Yes, androgen supplementation in elderly men improves libido, but there is a threshold level beyond which there is no further improvement of response.

Sexual satisfaction and fulfillment are based on the attitudes and behavior of a couple, not just on those of an individual. If enhancement of libido is an aging man's primary objective in considering androgen supplementation therapy, he must recognize that much (but not all) of the information on this subject is based on subjective data gathering, which is less quantitative than clinical or chemical measurements that document other physical benefits of such therapy. However, for those who select to enhance their androgen status to obtain these physical benefits, the effects on sexual attitudes and performance may bring additional satisfaction with androgen supplementation therapy.

20 • Can AST help brain function in aging men?

Cognitive function frequently declines with aging, so it is reasonable to suspect that the declining levels of testosterone in aging men may be a factor. Many scientific studies of an observational nature have been carried out to test this hypothesis. One way to approach this question is to determine whether an older man's testosterone level is correlated with his cognitive function. Do men who perform well on standard neuropsychological tests have higher circulating testosterone levels than men who perform poorly? Yes, it turns out that they do.

A group of researchers at the University of California-San Diego did an analysis of more than 500 men, 59–89 years of age. The subjects were noninstitutionalized residents of Rancho Bernardo, California. The investigators recorded the values of the men's total testosterone, and subsequently a battery of 12 standard neuropsychological tests were given that test memory, immediate and delayed recall, fluency, and several other cognitive functions. Although the association proved to be weak, they found that high total testosterone levels were predictive of better performance on several of the tests for cognitive function. Other investigators have confirmed this, fine-tuning their conclusions to emphasize the importance of bioavailable testosterone (the portion that is active in the body). A study of 300 men living near Pittsburgh found that there was no consistent correlation between total testosterone level and cognitive test scores, but men with high bioavailable testosterone performed better in all tests. This makes sense physiologically because it is more likely that biologically available hormone would be available to the brain and thus be more closely associated with central nervous system-controlled functions such as cognition.

To conclude that testosterone can affect the brain, you have to be reasonably sure that the hormone, in some active form, actually reaches the brain. This cannot be taken for granted because of a physiological phenomenon called the blood-brain barrier. The brain is protected by the blood-brain barrier from circulating elements that could be noxious or toxic to the delicate brain cells.

The brain is well oxygenated via the oxygen-carrying red blood cells, but there is a tight seal of cells that line the blood vessels. This acts as a barrier that keeps out almost everything except blood gases and small nutritional molecules. Does testosterone pass through the barrier? Indeed, it does, but only in the bioavailable form, unattached to the large carrier that binds most of the testosterone found in the blood and the major component of the total testosterone value in circulation. We can assume that the passage of free testosterone across the blood-brain barrier is possible because the cells in some regions of the brain possess androgen receptors, which are able to bind testosterone molecules that arrive via the bloodstream.

Observations of this nature suggest a next logical step: Can cognitive function be improved by giving testosterone supplementation therapy to older men with low levels of bioavailable testosterone? A group at the University of Washington Medical School in Seattle studied 25 men aged 50–80 years. The participants received either testosterone injections weekly or a placebo injection for six weeks. After the six weeks, the scientists measured the blood testosterone levels of the men and conducted a battery of neuropsychological tests. By the end of the treatment period, total circulating testosterone had been raised more than 100% and free testosterone levels also increased. The treated men had significant improvements in spatial memory (recall of a walking route), spatial ability (block construction), and verbal memory (recall of a short story), compared to the placebo group.

The researchers concluded that short-term testosterone treatment enhances cognitive function in healthy older men. This study confirms similar observations of earlier studies, whether the testosterone supplementation is given by injection or by another route. In fact, an even more recent study found an improvement in cognitive function using different tests when the testosterone was delivered via transdermal patch, one of the new forms of delivery.

Observational studies of this kind of men using AST are abundant and have produced impressive data. By late 2002, more than 200 publications on AST had appeared in the scientific literature. These studies provide strong evidence that AST, in the form of testosterone injections, gel, or patches, can cause improvement in positive mood and a decrease in negative moods during the trial period. One study carried out for six months reported that men who received testosterone treatment reported an increase in sense of well-being and an increase in energy and a decrease in negative mood parameters such as sadness and irritability. But the mood changes used do not necessarily reflect an influence of the hormone treatment on brain function directly.

It is a giant leap from mood changes to clear parameters of brain function. Maintaining mental function in old age is one of the greatest worries of the elderly, so any evidence of a beneficial treatment in this regard is enthusiastically embraced. The ability to use words and numbers accurately, the speed of information processing, and memory are specific brain functions that generally decline with aging. Can it be demonstrated that AST improves memory or any of these other specific cognitive functions? Using tests of mathematical reasoning and interpreting spatial relationships, researchers have found a strong correlation between testosterone levels in the blood of young, healthy men and good test performance.

This is encouraging for testosterone advocates, but the scientific literature has a lot of background noise that makes it difficult to know how much weight to put on this observation. For example, when older men with partial androgen deficiency were tested after three months of using a gel containing dihydrotestosterone, they failed to show an improvement in cognitive functions compared to men who had taken placebos. However, since the baseline scores for both the placebo group and the treatment group at the start of the trial were near the maximum, about all we can conclude from this is that AST for three months doesn't make normally smart men smarter.

Many additional studies using animal models have also been published. A study in mice, for example, found that androgens protect against cognitive deficits caused by factors similar to the cause of Alzheimer's disease in people. Basically, what the study shows is that reducing androgen receptor levels in the brain contributes to an Alzheimer-like cognitive decline in mice.

Several of the human studies describe observations that also pertain to Alzheimer's disease. At Oxford University, researchers at the Oxford Project to Investigate Memory and Ageing reported that a low testosterone level is potentially a risk factor for men who are genetically at risk of Alzheimer's disease. The same British group investigated 83 men with dementia of the Alzheimer's type and found that low total testosterone levels could exacerbate the disease. A study that demonstrates the biochemical pathway though which androgens given to aging men could prevent or delay Alzheimer's disease was published in the *Proceedings of the National Academy of Sciences*.

In spite of the encouraging observational findings, we have to conclude that there are not sufficient data to support the use of testosterone (or DHEA, which has also been described as being effective) for the treatment of depression, other mood changes, memory deficits, or other cognitive functions.

It would be difficult to prove the relationship between androgen supplementation and brain function without a shadow of a doubt. An ideal study design would be to randomly assign older men to two groups, one receiving androgen supplementation therapy, the other receiving a placebo. All men would have to be matched for many factors that might influence the result: age, education, diet, exercise habits, smoking, medications used, family history, and several others. At the end of the prospective study, say 10 years, each subject would be evaluated for cognitive function and for signs of the onset of Alzheimer's disease. Deciding what tests to perform might be easy to agree on, but what about the AST to be used in the study? Would the use of one type of AST, such as a testosterone gel, indicate what to expect from any other supplementation therapy? The cost of such a study would be enormous and, in the end, the results might be questionable since all influencing factors would be hard to control.

The National Institutes of Health considered funding a trial like this that would have been a 6-year trial with 6000 men but dropped the idea when the substantial cost became apparent. It would have cost more than $100 million, and the chances are it would never be carried to completion because of drop-out rates and other reasons. However, NIH has requested the U.S. Institute of Medicine to evaluate the need for and feasibility of a prospective study of testosterone supplementation therapy in aging men.

It is rare for any prescription drug to have this kind of information to back up claims for safety and effectiveness. In fact, the only such study of this nature to evaluate the risks and benefits of aspirin, planned to last for 20 years, was abruptly halted after only 4 years. By then it was obvious that aspirin was protecting men from heart attacks, so it would have been unethical to continue giving some men only aspirin-free placebos and depriving them of the established benefit of aspirin that had already been proven. On the other hand, what did the study prove about the long-term risk of hemorrhagic stroke? Unfortunately, it was not carried out long enough to reach a definitive conclusion. If the FDA required long-term prospective studies of this type before a drug could be approved for marketing, we would probably have no new drug therapies.

Tantalizing as it may seem, the use of testosterone supplementation therapy to improve brain function or to delay the onset of Alzheimer's disease is not warranted on the basis of information currently available. If men choose to use AST for other symptoms of andropause, a beneficial effect on cognition should not be high on the list of expectations.

III • • • Questions and Answers

• • • Questions about menopause

Why do women have menopause?

Women have menopause because their ovaries cease functioning. Estrogen and progesterone production by the ovaries becomes erratic, and the total amounts of hormones produced dramatically decrease. The uterine lining depends on estrogen and progesterone for the monthly buildup leading to menstruation, so when these ovarian hormones are no longer present, the menstrual flow no longer occurs. Periods usually become irregular at first, but they can cease abruptly.

At what age does menopause occur?

The age at which menopause occurs varies from person to person. The average age of menopause in the United States is 51, but the range that is considered normal is from age 42 to 58. The process is almost always complete by age 55.

What are the signs of menopause?

The principal sign is variation in the menstrual pattern, ending in complete cessation of periods. Bodily changes occur as a result of the absence of the ovarian hormones. One of the earliest signs of estrogen deficiency is hot flashes which, in extreme cases, can be debilitating. Hot flashes occur in most menopausal women but some women have none at all. The flashes are associated with flushing of the face, an overwhelming feeling of bodily heat, and perspiration. Hot flashes can cause night sweats and sleep deprivation. Somewhat later in the symptom sequence, there may be vaginal dryness and failure to lubricate during sexual stimulation. There may also be urinary symptoms due to thinning of the vaginal wall supporting the bladder.

What is hormone replacement therapy (HRT)?

Hormone replacement therapy (HRT) refers to the use of hormones to replace those produced by the ovaries before menopause. The term is not really accurate, so we have chosen not to use it in this book. A better term, recommended by the FDA, is "menopausal hormone therapy." HRT or HT is the term applied when estrogen is used in combination with a progesteronelike compound (progestin). A progestin is added to the estrogen to prevent overstimulation of the cells that line the uterus (the endometrium), which can result in precancerous changes or even endometrial cancer.

What is estrogen replacement therapy?

Estrogen replacement therapy (ERT or ET) refers to the use of estrogen alone for the management of menopausal symptoms. ET is used for women who have had a hysterectomy so that uterine cancer is no longer possible. Since there is no uterus, bleeding irregularities are not an issue when ET is used.

Why should women consider HT?

HT provides the most efficient treatment of hot flashes, night sweats, sleep disturbances, and mood changes associated with menopause. It also protects the vagina, preserving sexual function, and has a positive effect on maintaining bone strength. The downside of HT must be considered. With long-term use of HT, the absolute risk of breast cancer is increased at a magnitude of about 8 additional cases per 10,000 women per year. There is also an increased risk for thromboembolic disease at about the same scale: annual risk rates of about one-tenth of 1%.

At what age should a woman consider whether to start HT?

Once a woman has developed symptoms that signal she is either peri-menopausal or menopausal, it is time to consider some form of HT. For the perimenopausal woman with irregular menses who is still sporadically ovulating, low-dose oral contraceptives are a reasonable approach. Women who are well past menopause can continue HT if withdrawal of treatment brings on a return of their symptoms. If the problem is vaginal dryness and urinary symptoms, a woman can use some form of HT well into old age, adjusting dosage and route of administration. Older women should consider using vaginal estrogen, or possibly an estrogen/progestin combination delivered by dermal patch.

Once started, is HT used for the rest of a woman's life?

Starting HT should never commit a woman to continue it indefinitely. Overall health status should be evaluated at least yearly. The annual visit allows a review of health issues that may not be related to menopause. At the time of the annual visit, alternative treatment can be considered. If the principal reason for initiating the HT was severe menopausal symptoms, gradual withdrawal of the HT may show that the treatment is no longer required. A woman who has been on HT for three or more years for whom sexual function is an important issue may wish to discontinue the HT and substitute a vaginal estrogen. When there is evidence of bone loss, non-hormonal management of bone health can be substituted for HT.

What options do women have in selecting HT, and how should the selection be made?

A wide variety of HT approaches are available. In addition to FDA-approved products, phytoestrogens, herbal products, and various food supplements are sold in health food stores. A decision as to which HT is finally used should be individualized. For severe hot flashes the first choice is an oral combination of estrogen and progestin, or a transdermal patch containing estrogen and progestin. The choice of one over another is a matter of personal preference. Women who have had hysterectomies can use estrogen only, and they have a wide variety of options. A number of oral estrogen preparations are available. There is an estrogen skin patch, a slow-release vaginal ring, and vaginal tablets or creams which have a local effect with minimal absorption.

How widely used is HT in the United States?

About 20% of America's 40 million women of menopausal age in 2002 used HT. The most widely used products on the HT market are the Premarin products including the popular single-pill formulation Prempro. This pill combines conjugated equine estrogens with a progestin. The July 2002 news coverage of the Women's Health Initiative study caused a sharp drop in Prempro prescriptions, but three months later the Premarin products retained almost 70% of the estrogen/progestin market. Other FDA-approved estrogen/progestin combinations make up the balance.

What are SERMS and why are they important in the menopause?

SERM stands for selective estrogen receptor modulator. As its name implies, a SERM is designed to act selectively on some estrogen receptors, causing only the tissues affected to respond. Other estrogen receptors are not affected, and these tissues fail to react at all. An ideal SERM for menopause would be one which would have a positive effect on menopausal symptoms, including hot flashes and vaginal dryness, as well as an effect on the other important estrogen-reactive tissues, such as the bone and the brain, while having no effect or even a blocking effect on the receptors of the breast and endometrium. The currently available SERMS do not satisfy all of these criteria. For example, raloxifene (Evista) exerts a positive effect on the bone, a minimal effect on the endometrium, and a protective effect on the breast, but it does nothing for hot flashes or vaginal dryness.

Will SERMS control hot flashes?

As stated above, the currently available SERMS do not control hot flashes; they make them worse. A woman who is experiencing debilitating hot flashes would not be satisfied with the SERMs currently available, in spite of the positive effect on bone and a protective effect on breast tissue. There are new SERMs in the research pipeline that may also provide relief from hot flashes in addition to their other beneficial effects. Or, they may be used with an estrogen to provide relief from vasomotor symptoms.

Should androgens (testosterone) be used with HT for women?

The main indication for the use of testosterone is to improve sexual function. When oral estrogen is combined with an orally active androgen (methyltestosterone), it is still necessary to use a progestational agent in women who have a uterus. The woman who has had her ovaries and uterus removed before natural menopause should consider the use of an estrogen/testosterone combination, since the testosterone level falls sharply after the surgery.

Are herbal products useful for menopause?

With few exceptions, the herbal products that are marketed for menopausal symptoms have not been rigorously tested in scientifically valid studies. Many of these have side effects and even dangerous interactions with other medications. For example, St. John's wort, a popular herbal product, reduces the effectiveness of oral contraceptives. A standardized alcoholic extract of black cohosh, a plant root marketed as Remifemin, has been shown in some studies to reduce hot flashes and other menopausal symptoms, but other studies have failed to confirm this. For the remainder of the numerous products available, evidence for their effectiveness is largely anecdotal.

Do women have more depression with menopause?

Depression can occur during times when estrogen levels are low (e.g., after childbirth). There is a tendency toward depression during the menopausal adjustment, which is also a period of estrogen deprivation. However, because menopause often occurs at an age when other changes in a woman's life could cause mental stress, it is difficult to separate out symptoms that are triggered by life situations from those that are more directly the result of changing hormones.

Will severe untreated hot flashes lead to brain damage?

Hot flashes can be debilitating, especially when they interfere with sleep. Patients sometimes express anxiety over the long-term impact of hot flashes on brain function. The typical question is, "Am I going crazy, and if this continues will it do any permanent damage?" The answer is an unequivocal no. In the majority of cases, even when untreated, hot flashes are self-limiting. Furthermore, there are no known mechanisms associated with the production of hot flashes that could cause brain damage.

Does menopause cause women to gain weight?

Yes, but weight gain is not inevitable. Weight gain depends on the balance between calories consumed and calories expended and the body's efficiency in utilizing calories. Older women tend to lead a more sedentary life. Added to this, there tends to be a change in eating habits leading to higher total calories consumed. Furthermore, with age the body metabolizes calories more frugally so that less food is required. The net result of this calorie increase and conservation is fat storage and increased weight. There is also a changing distribution of fat. The adipose cells in the buttocks, waist, and torso tend to store this additional fat.

Does HT influence weight gain?

The influence of HT on weight gain in menopause has been extensively investigated. Women randomly assigned to HT and to no-treatment groups have an equivalent weight gain. Nevertheless, many patients in my practice are convinced that they have gained weight directly as a result of estrogen treatment and insist that it seemed easier to take the weight off before they were treated or when the hormones are discontinued. Weight control serves to emphasize the importance of promoting a healthy lifestyle that includes limited caloric intake, an appropriately balanced diet, and a daily exercise program.

Does menopause cause a change in body composition and contour?

Almost invariably, women experience a change in weight distribution and body composition with the onset of menopause. The percentage of body fat increases while muscle and bone weights decrease. Body contour alterations add inches to the waistline and flanks, and frequently increase breast size.

Can women who have had endometriosis use ET if they have had a hysterectomy?

The one exception to the use of estrogen alone in women without a uterus is in case a woman has a history of severe endometriosis. In these cases, remnants of endometrium may still be present in the abdomen even after hysterectomy and other surgery for the condition. These remnants could be stimulated excessively and painfully with estrogen alone therapy. Hence, the addition of a progestin is advised.

Can HT prevent Alzheimer's disease and memory loss?

Estrogen has a direct effect on the brain. Regions of the brain contain estrogen receptors, providing the mechanism to respond to estrogen. There is suggestive evidence of some improvement in memory in women who are on HT or ET, but additional clinical studies are warranted before firm claims can be made. Evidence is accumulating that estrogen does have a positive effect on the brain's ability to handle stress and on cognitive function in general. The issue as to whether Alzheimer's disease can be prevented or delayed remains unresolved but is under study.

Does HT help prevent heart attacks and strokes?

Observational studies over many years suggested that HT prevents heart attacks, but this has not been substantiated. The fact that HT/ET has a beneficial effect on the lipid profile considered to be preventive against atherosclerosis reinforced this idea. This is because heart attacks result mainly from the accumulation of lipid plaques in the coronary arteries. The same reasoning was applied to explain why HT might protect against strokes. The placebo-controlled study of the Women's Health Initiative has not substantiated that the heart is protected by the beneficial changes in blood lipid pattern. To the contrary, there was increased risk of an adverse reaction including both heart attack and stroke in women using estrogen and progestin therapy.

Is there a greater risk of clotting and pulmonary embolus with HT?

There is a somewhat increased risk of thrombosis and its consequence, pulmonary embolism, in women using HT/ET. This was also a finding of the WHI study. Women with a history of a blood-clot event should not use HT.

Should women with high cholesterol use HT?

There is definite evidence that HT/ET improves the cholesterol profile. Low-density lipoprotein (LDL), the bad cholesterol, decreases, and high-density lipoprotein (HDL), the good cholesterol, increases. Hence, high cholesterol is not a contraindication for the use of HT. Improving the cholesterol profile with HT, however, does not result in a reduced risk of cardiovascular adverse events.

Does HT prevent bone loss and osteoporosis associated with aging?

HT helps maintain bone mineral density. The maximal benefit appears to be obtained with three years of HT use. Consequently, it prevents osteoporosis and lowers the incidence of hip and vertebral fractures substantially. Other nonhormonal treatments are available that exert a nearly equal effect on bone.

What happens to bone density when a woman stops using HT?

There is not a rapid loss of bone minerals when a woman stops using HT. Her bone density declines at the same rate as women who have not used HT: about 1% during the first year and about half that in the ensuing years.

What is the impact of HT on diabetes?

There is no firm information to suggest that there is either a positive or negative effect of HT on diabetes. Because diabetics tend to have higher cholesterol levels than nondiabetics, the cholesterol-altering properties of HT might be a benefit.

Does HT have a cosmetic effect on the skin?

Many women who are on HT are convinced that there is a positive cosmetic effect on both the tone and consistency of skin. They may be right because skin cells do contain estrogen receptors. Nevertheless, there is no scientific information to back up the claim that HT prevents wrinkles. Claims that estrogen-containing creams improve skin tone have not been proven, either.

Does HT cause or prevent thinning hair?

There are no firm studies which point in either direction. Some women report hair loss and others report hair growth once they are on HT or ET.

In any case, there is no scientific evidence to recommend HT or ET for hair loss management.

Does HT or ET affect varicose veins?

There is no evidence that varicose veins are significantly affected by HT or ET. We know that varicose veins tend to increase in number and severity in pregnancy, and it was believed that this is an estrogen effect. This is not the case; there are many other factors involved. Since varicosities are associated with aging generally, they certainly occur independent of estrogen.

Does HT have an effect on teeth or gums?

The positive effect of HT/ET on total bone composition is well established, and some studies suggest that HT prevents or delays the jaw bone regression that can occur in aging women. When no treatment is used to maintain bone strength, aging itself has a negative effect on teeth and gums.

Can HT help prevent loss of sight or hearing with age?

There is no evidence that HT has any effect on decline in visual and hearing acuity with age. Women with hearing impairment should be encouraged to seek the benefits of modern hearing aids and to improve vision with corrective lenses.

Will HT prevent watery eyes in the elderly?

Tears are a product of the lacrimal glands and are released via the lacrimal ducts. These contain estrogen receptors, but the effect of estrogen replacement on their function has not been established by scientific evidence.

Can a woman use ET if she has had breast cancer?

Physicians are reluctant to treat any woman with estrogen when there is a history of breast cancer. To establish a diagnosis of breast cancer, a biopsy is evaluated. In a woman with severe, uncontrollable hot flashes who has had breast cancer that did not contain estrogen receptors, it would be reasonable to attempt to relieve her symptoms with a limited course of a low dose of estrogen. When the breast cancer is estrogen-receptor positive, however, it would certainly be unwise to use a medication with the potential of stimulating further growth. The SERMs tamoxifen and raloxifene are recommended in treatment of estrogen-sensitive breast cancers inasmuch as both cause tumor regression. They have the added advantage of providing bone protection, although they are associated with an increased risk of thromboembolic disease and do not control vasomotor symptoms such as hot flashes.

Does adding a progestin have any effect on breast cancer risk?

We do not know whether there is an additive breast cancer risk when a progestin is added. The Women's Health Initiative study was discontinued when it was noted that there were 8 additional cases of breast cancer per 10,000 women per year in the HT (Prempro)-treated group. A companion study using estrogen alone, started at the same time, was allowed to continue, but the final results will not be available for at least two years. This raises the suspicion, yet to be proven, that the progestin may be responsible for the added risk. There is no evidence, as was previously believed, that progestin provides a protective effect against breast cancer.

Can a woman use HT/ET if her mother suffered from breast cancer?

A woman in the high-risk category has at least two first-degree (mother or sister) or two second-degree (cousin or aunt) relatives in whom breast cancer was diagnosed before age 60. A woman whose mother but no other relative has had breast cancer is not considered high risk unless her mother developed the cancer before age 40. Anyone whose mother has had breast cancer, whatever the age, is a candidate for careful surveillance with serious attention to periodic mammograms and self-examination. Since the discovery of the breast cancer genes, *BRCA*-1 and *BRCA*-2, the debate has continued as to how this information should be used. It is unlikely that there will ever be an HT study of a group of patients who have these genes. Nevertheless, it seems intuitive that it would be inappropriate to consider HT or ET use in women who already have a genetic risk factor for breast cancer.

Does menopause mean an end to fertility?

Once a woman is clearly menopausal, which implies that ovulation has ceased entirely, fertility is no longer an option. The availability of sophisticated assisted reproductive technologies has, however, made postmenopausal pregnancy possible, but only with the use of donor eggs. In the perimenopausal interval, ovulation can occur sporadically. This carries the remote possibility of pregnancy. With age, the quality of the eggs declines, further diminishing the likelihood of a pregnancy. The perimenopausal woman with irregular menstrual periods should consider short-term use of a low-dose oral contraceptive which would regularize the periods, and at the same time provide contraceptive protection.

Can HT maintain libido and sexual satisfaction for menopausal women?

HT is useful in maintaining the flexibility and thickness of the vaginal wall, allowing vaginal intercourse to continue. The decline in estrogen levels associated with menopause results in thinning of the vagina, and there may be pain with intercourse. Estrogen can reverse this process entirely. In some women, especially those whose ovaries were surgically removed before natural menopause, libido may be impaired because of the loss of the androgen normally produced by the ovaries. In these cases the addition of testosterone to the HT regimen can enhance libido.

How should women handle contraception as they approach menopause?

Until ovulation has completely ceased, one cannot be sure that pregnancy will not occur. Fertility is markedly diminished in the perimenopausal interval, however, and the likelihood of pregnancy is small. The use of low-dose oral contraception is a reasonable choice, especially in women who continue to ovulate irregularly.

What is the effect of hormones on ovarian, uterine, and breast cancer?

There is a vast literature on the relationship between HT/ET and cancer of the breast and of the reproductive tract. Some of it is contradictory. Epidemiological data have established an increased risk of breast cancer associated with HT, but the data are not definitive concerning ET. Women who use for ET 10 years or longer may be at increased risk of ovarian cancer. Women who use hormones as oral contraceptives are protected against ovarian cancer.

Can HT protect against colon cancer?

There is a protective effect of HT against colorectal cancer. In the largest prospective controlled study carried out to date, the Women's Health

Initiative study, there were 6 fewer cases of colon cancer per 10,000 women years of use. This is a 40% decline in the rate found among a comparable group of women taking a placebo pill. This benefit, however, is no substitute for colonoscopic examinations at a frequency depending on age and family history.

Do different races/ethnic groups experience menopause differently?

Differences have been detected in racial groups. For example, Japanese women appear to have a lower incidence of menopausal symptoms, including hot flashes. This may be more the result of the Japanese diet, which is high in soy proteins containing phytoestrogens, than of genetics. It has been suggested that menopausal symptoms occur less frequently in African-American women, but this has not been substantiated.

Do different races/ethnic groups respond to HT differently?

There is no evidence that there is a racial difference in response to HT. There are subtle differences in the estrogen receptors in some women that modify response to estrogen, but these genetic differences have not been identified as being racially related. There are wide variations in attitude toward menopause from one ethnic group to another.

I am now menopausal, and after months of debilitating hot flashes I am at my wit's end. I have read about risks of HT but I would like to try it not only because of hot flashes but also because of my inability to sleep. What will help me with this decision?

The importance of controlling hot flashes and sleep disturbances should not be underestimated, and HT still provides the most efficient and effective approach to these symptoms. The American College of Obstetricians and Gynecologists recommends that HT be used at the lowest dose for the shortest time that works for the individual woman with regular, at least yearly, consultations to review the decision to remain on HT.

What if, after a decision to discontinue HT, the menopausal symptoms return with severity?

Women who have been on HT for many years sometimes stop only to find that menopausal symptoms recur. Many decide to resume HT for as long as is necessary, using the lowest dose that will control the symptoms. This is a wise decision. Lifestyle modifications, such as eliminating smoking, caffeine, and alcohol; regular exercise; and finding ways to reduce stress levels can sometimes help.

Two years ago my physician prescribed HT, taking into account a strong family history of heart disease and my own unfavorable lipid profile. Should I continue to use HT?

HT does not prevent heart disease in healthy women, nor does it protect women who have preexisting heart disease. In fact, HT may be associated with a slight increase in the chances of angina or a heart attack. If HT was prescribed primarily to prevent heart disease, it should be discontinued and consideration given to using other measures for lowering cholesterol, such as the use of statins along with blood pressure monitoring, and healthy lifestyles, including diet modification and a program of regular exercise. There is no substitute for good cardiac care.

The HT arm of the Women's Health Initiative study was discontinued, but the portion of the study which used estrogen alone was not. Does this suggest that estrogen without progestin is safer, and, if so, should women on HT switch to ET?

The women in the study who were treated with estrogen alone all had had hysterectomies. Women with an intact uterus should not use unopposed estrogen because of the increased risk of overstimulation of the uterine lining, resulting in hyperplasia and in some cases, frank cancer. Both HT and ET continue to be accepted approaches to menopausal management, but ET is reserved only for those women who have had hysterectomies.

Since the Women's Health Initiative study reported on the use of the estrogen/progestin combination, Prempro, would it not be reasonable to switch to an estrogen/progestin combination using other hormones?

The findings of the Women's Health Initiative study can be applied only to the Prempro formulation, at the dose of 0.625 mg of conjugated equine estrogens combined with 2.5 mg of medroxyprogesterone acetate. There is no way of knowing whether other doses or other hormonal regimens will be found to be safer, nor are they at this point the subject of such an extensive prospective placebo-controlled trial. There is no scientific basis for switching from Prempro to another estrogen/progestin combination.

Would it be safer to use a combination of "natural" hormones produced by the human body?

"Naturalness" does not endow a hormone with the ability to select in a beneficial way the cells with which it will interact. Regardless of the source of a hormone, it exerts it biological effects, both favorable and unfavorable, because it interacts with specialized receptors on target cells. This is where SERMs come in because they are designed to have selective action on some tissues and not others, with the goal of improving safety.

Is there a simple way for a woman to decide if the risks of HT outweigh the benefits for her?

There is no checklist that can give you a foolproof answer. Women should realize that there is a big difference in risk analysis between short-term use of HT and long-term use. Short-term use carries minimal risk and is highly effective in reducing or eliminating hot flashes, night sweats, vaginal dryness, and other bodily changes that diminish a woman's quality of life. The documented long-term risks of HT which include modest increases in breast cancer, coronary heart disease, stroke, and blood clots are serious and merit concern. These need to be weighed against some proven long-term benefits including a substantially lower risk of osteoporosis and hip or vertebral fractures, and a lower risk of colorectal cancer, as well as the short-term benefits of controlling hot flashes and other menopausal symptoms.

What is the final message on HT for menopausal women?

There can be no final message because research is still continuing, and we learn more every month. Our knowledge might best be divided as "pre-Women's Health Initiative (WHI)" and "post-WHI." Before the results of the WHI study were released in July 2002, we knew that HT is unmatched for controlling menopausal symptoms and, like other medications, could hold off the hazards of osteoporosis. Post-WHI we still know all of this is true. Before WHI we were aware that these benefits come with a risk of some increase in the chance of developing breast cancer after long-term use, even though the risk of death due to breast cancer does not increase among HT users. After WHI we have a confirmation of both of these facts with the annual increase measured to be one-tenth of 1%. That precise measurement of risk is new and stands at least until another study is complete. Before WHI the assertions that HT could prevent heart disease or protect against a second heart attack had been debunked by other studies. After WHI we can be certain of this and, in fact, alert women that HT carries the risk of an increase in some cardio-vascular-related adverse reactions. Again, the annual increase for all adverse events in this category combined is a fraction of 1%. The take-home message is that there are both benefits and risks. There is no single answer for every woman when it comes to deciding on HT.

• • • Questions about andropause

Is there a man's equivalent to a woman's menopause?

Not exactly, but many men experience aging changes similar to some of the changes of a woman's menopause. They tend to lose muscle mass and strength and gain abdominal fat. Their bones lose density because of calcium depletion so that they can develop osteoporosis or the less severe degree of the condition known as osteopenia. Men do not experience hot flashes as they age, but mood changes, memory loss, and impairment of other brain cognitive functions are not different from the experience of aging women. Unlike the female menopause, which is part of women's genetic constitution, this set of changes is not predestined to happen to all men. A man's testes can keep working throughout his lifetime but, with aging, the function of the testes may become impaired because of aging conditions that block blood supply to either the testes or the pituitary gland or interfere with nerve systems.

Are "partial androgen deficiency," "male climacteric," "male menopause," and "andropause" all different terms for the same thing?

Yes, and each phrase has its limitations. The most appropriate is "partial androgen deficiency," but the term is rarely used by the general public. The term "andropause" is fairly accurate and has gained wider acceptance. Strictly speaking, the male's androgen production does not end but diminishes.

Why don't we hear much about andropause and androgen supplementation therapy?

The media are beginning to discover andropause, so you can expect to read and hear more about it. Since good news seems not to be as newsworthy as bad news, you'll probably begin to hear about the uncertainties of androgen supplementation therapy more than the benefits. There has already been a front page *New York Times* article (August 19, 2002) titled "Male Hormone Therapy Popular But Untested" that reported on the absence of a long-term epidemiological study but ignored the literally hundreds of articles in scientific journals on the subject. Another reason for the relative silence is that until Androgel, a gel applied to the skin, the products available for hormone replacement during andropause had deficiencies that did not encourage their use so that treatment of andropause was limited.

Is there a safe androgen supplementation therapy for men?

The term we prefer for male hormone therapy in aging is androgen supplementation therapy (AST). Many FDA-approved products for AST have been available for years and have been used mainly for the treatment of clinical conditions resulting in inadequate testicular function (hypogonadism) in young men. Since 1999, a testosterone-releasing gel (Androgel) has been marketed as a prescription drug. This has changed the landscape. The gel is growing in popularity in the United States and is widely used in other countries. Androgel is FDA-approved for use by men suffering complaints derived from androgen deficiency, which means that doctors can comfortably prescribe Androgel for the androgen deficiency of aging males as well as for clinical hypogonadism.

Do you take AST?

We each looked into it and found that our testosterone levels are not below normal so that supplementation was not called for. In any event, our medical histories are such that we would not be good candidates for testosterone supplementation therapy, but when the first designer androgen now being tested (MENT) comes on the market, we'll gladly consider using it.

Is testosterone the only male hormone normally produced in the body?

No, and testosterone is not even the most potent. Both the testis and the adrenal gland produce testosterone by converting cholesterol into various androgenic molecules, and there are other androgens derived from the conversion of testosterone into other compounds as part of the body's normal metabolism. One of these metabolites is dihydrotestosterone, which is two and a half times as potent as testosterone and is found in far higher concentration in the prostate gland than is testosterone.

What do athletes take to build muscles and improve their performance?

That's a good question but hard to answer. Athletes do not like to talk about their use of steroids ("'roids," as they are frequently referred to in the locker room) but the volume of sales of products touted as muscle builders is huge. Athletes and body builders tend to "stack" the use of dietary supplements, taking very large doses of several androgens at the same time. Among the most popular are androstendione and dehydro-epiandrosterone (DHEA), both marketed as dietary supplements without close FDA surveillance. In some sports, athletes take human growth hormone (hGH) for muscle building and other hormonelike compounds that intensify synthesis of red blood cells so that they have more oxygen-carrying capacity and higher endurance.

Is loss of libido with aging normal for men?

Yes, but it is not inevitable. In a study we did on aging and hormones, many men in their 80s had enough libido to try to grope the nurses in the urology ward where they were patients. There is more scientific evidence based on surveys indicating that libido loss with aging is individual.

Can AST prevent libido loss?

Several studies have reported good results using AST to prevent or reverse the loss of libido in older men. AST, however, does not affect impotence caused by erectile dysfunction.

Can men prevent Alzheimer's disease or memory loss by taking hormones?

This is not proven, although there have been claims to this effect. AST should not be considered as treatment for Alzheimer's because there is no supportive evidence that it can reverse the disease. The limited information available pertains to the possibility that AST may delay the onset of Alzheimer's disease.

What is the effect of AST on the prostate?

Androgens can cause an increase in prostate size and could accelerate the growth of preexisting cancer cells. This is the main reason for hesitancy in using AST. The culprit, however, is not testosterone itself, but the potent metabolite to which it can be converted, dihydrotestosterone (DHT). As long as testosterone levels are kept within normal limits and good prostate surveillance is maintained (annual check-ups with prostate-specific antigen determinations), AST can be considered prostate safe.

Does AST increase the risk for other types of cancer?

There is no evidence that androgen increases the risk of other cancers, even if given in supranormal amounts. Because estrogen is an important conversion product of testosterone, breast cancer in men is a theoretical possibility. However, this has never been reported in the scientific literature as a side effect of AST.

Can AST increase the risk of heart or vascular problems?

Testosterone has always had a reputation of being bad for the heart, but the opposite may be true. Many studies find that the lipid profile changes in a heart-friendly direction when men are using AST. The level of low-density lipoprotein, the bad cholesterol, goes down, and the ratio of good to bad cholesterol improves. Thus, there is solid evidence that for one of the conditions of cardiovascular disease, plaque formation in the blood vessels, AST can be beneficial. Androgens have also been shown to maintain blood vessel flexibility by preventing the changes that lead to arteriosclerosis (hardening of the arteries). Adverse effects of AST on the heart, however, may be of a different nature. The question cannot be answered satisfactorily until there is a properly designed prospective study that monitors the cardiovascular status of men on AST compared with matched controls. Androstendione can lower blood levels of higher-density lipoprotein cholesterol. This is not good for heart health.

Does AST affect the blood?

AST can cause an increase in the production of red blood cells so that the blood becomes more concentrated. That's good news and bad news. The good news is that the result of a higher hematocrit (the measure of red blood cell concentration) is a higher oxygen-carrying capacity. The bad news is that clotting potential is enhanced, and this could lead to a stroke or blot clot in the lung. Another beneficial effect on the blood is enhancing the immune system so that infection-fighting cells (immuno-potential cells) are replaced more rapidly and are more abundant.

Does AST have an effect on weight gain or fat distribution for older men?

Remodeling of body fat distribution can be expected with AST. Abdominal fat is reduced and, depending on an accompanying exercise routine, the body contour can be changed dramatically. Weight gain can occur if muscle mass is being built up at the same time, so the net result is a shift in weight from the proportion that is fat and the proportion that is muscle and bone.

Do men taking AST have breast enlargement?

Overdosing with androgens will definitely cause breast enlargement because androgens are converted to estrogen in the body, and these estrogens can stimulate breast tissue growth. If testosterone levels are kept within a normal range, this is no more a risk than a man has with natural testosterone levels. Some dietary supplements used by body-builders are androgens that are rapidly converted to estrogens, causing breast enlargement.

Can men maintain muscle mass and bone density with AST?

These are probably the most carefully studied end results of AST, so that it can be fully documented that the answer is yes. There are studies in which men have been followed for three years using AST and compared to others who were given placebos. The beneficial effect with respect to increase muscle mass and bone mineral density is clear cut.

Can AST prevent vision changes?

There have been claims that AST helps maintain lens flexibility and slows down cataract formation. These observational studies cannot be taken as proof, however. There is no substitute for good vision care.

Can hormone therapy help men with sleep disorders?

According to survey studies, the answer is yes. Men on AST report that they sleep better and feel more rested after a night's sleep. A conflicting finding is that men on AST have an increased frequency of sleep apnea (interrupted breathing patterns sometimes causing loud snoring). Sleep apnea usually causes interrupted sleep. Nevertheless, the number of reports of improved sleep outweighs the theoretical conclusion that sleep may be being disturbed by increased frequency of sleep apnea.

Can AST reduce fat in older men?

Not only can abdominal fat be reduced by using AST, but overall body fat can be reduced. The amount of fat loss and the time it takes to lose body fat depends on diet and exercise habits. Couch potatoes taking AST will continue to be couch potatoes.

Will AST prevent erectile dysfunction?

Testosterone deficiency is not ordinarily the cause of erectile dysfunction. Erectile dysfunction is caused by vascular changes that make it difficult for the penis to remain tumescent even when there is sexual arousal. The drug that has proven to be effective, silfenidine (Viagra) works through a totally different mechanism than stimulating androgen production. AST will not prevent erectile dysfunction.

What treatment options do men have for AST?

The prescription products approved by the FDA for androgen supplementation therapy are based on testosterone supplementation. Products are available that deliver testosterone by injection, by oral pill, by skin patch, or by skin gel. The gel product is by far the most popular. There is also a gel available in Europe that delivers the high-potency androgen DHT, but this is not approved for use by the FDA. Nonprescription products are available in nutritional supplement stores and via the internet. These nutritional supplements usually contain DHEA, DHEAS, or androstendione. Because they are classified as nutritional supplements they do not have to meet stringent FDA requirements concerning claims of effectiveness and safety.

Many men use nutritional supplements, like androstenedione or DHEA. Do they work?

There is a $2 billion market in the United States alone on muscle-building nutritional supplements. Looking at the bodies of many athletes and body-builders, obviously something is working. However, when scientific studies have tried to establish the effectiveness of products like DHEA (dihydroepiandrosterone) or androstenedione, they come up with negative results. So who is right, America's scientists or the country's body-builders? The problem is that while the scientific studies have been done using the recommended doses, actual use far exceeds these doses. This is because of "stacking," which is the practice of taking several andro-genic products at the same time. The doses used are huge and may be exceeding by far a safe level.

What are SARMs?

SARMs are selective androgen receptor modifiers. They are to androgens what SERMs are to estrogens. They are designer androgens synthesized by chemists to have some androgenic effects and not others. The mole-cule can achieve this by selectively interacting with androgen receptors on some cells but not on others. The ideal SARM, for example, might be one that has all the desirable effects of an androgen in maintaining bone density and muscle mass and strength, preventing the deposition of ab-dominal fat, and exerting any of the positive effects on brain function believed to be a possible bonus benefit of AST. At the same time, it would be prostate neutral and have no deleterious effects on the blood, liver, or cardiovascular conditions.

Why is MENT considered a promising advance for AST?

MENT comes close to meeting the definition of an ideal SARM. Because of its chemical structure, the body cannot convert it to DHT, the super-androgen responsible for prostate stimulation. At the same time, MENT exerts a testosteronelike muscle-building effect. If this promise holds up in clinical trials now under way, MENT could become an important prod-uct for AST. It would probably be marketed either as a long-acting im-plant or as a gel for daily application.

What is the final message on AST in andropause?

Men who believe they are losing muscle mass and strength, acquiring unwanted abdominal fat, losing interest in sex, tiring easily, becoming irritable, and suffering from depression or other mood changes should consider AST. The first step is to determine if your blood level of bioavailable testosterone is below normal. If it is within the normal range, don't expect to use medication to become "more normal." Consider weight loss, exercise, and other changes in lifestyle to improve your quality of life. If you are testosterone deficient, AST, monitored by your physician, is a sensible option, provided the therapy used maintains your free testosterone values within the range of normal and does not become supraphysiological. The risk–benefit ratio stays favorable as long as testosterone levels are not elevated above normal. Do not succumb to the idea that if a little is good, more must be better.

• • • Glossary of terms

adrenal gland. A gland above the kidney that produces cortisonelike hormones in response to stress and produces male-type hormones (androgens) that can be converted to estrogen elsewhere in the body.

alendronate. One of the biphosphonate group of drugs that preserve bone mineral density.

alkylated testosterone derivatives. Man-made derivatives of testosterone carrying a large (alkyl) side chain that makes testosterone orally active but can cause liver toxicity.

amenorrhea. The condition of a woman not having menstrual cycles.

androgens. Hormones that stimulate male sex characteristics.

androgen supplementation therapy. AST; the preferred term to describe hormone therapy for aging men.

andrology. The medical specialty pertaining to diagnosis and treatment of reproductive system disorders in men and boys.

androstenedione. A weak androgen that the body produces and converts into testosterone.

antioxidants. Substances that prevent a chemical byproduct of cellular metabolism (free radicals) from damaging DNA and perhaps causing cancer.

aphrodisiac. A substance believed to stimulate sexual interest.

aromatase. The enzyme that converts testosterone to an estrogen, a normal and important function.

arteriosclerosis. Hardening of the arteries due to the deposition of calcium in the walls, which reduces the vessel's flexibility; sometimes used interchangeably with atherosclerosis.

AST. See *androgen supplementation therapy.*

atherosclerosis. Narrowing of arteries due to the formation of lipid (fat) plaques on the inner wall. Lowering cholesterol levels in the blood reduces the chances of plaque formation.

atresia. The spontaneous loss of follicles within the ovary. It accounts for the disappearance of most of the ovary's follicles.

atrophy. Deterioration of a tissue when it lacks the stimulation of a hormone required for normal function or because of some other pathological condition.

Ayurvedic medicine. The ancient art of medicine described in the Indian Vedas (the world's oldest written record) and still practiced in India.

beta-amyloid. A protein that forms plaques in the brain believed to be responsible for Alzheimer's disease.

bioavailable testosterone. The portion of the circulating total testosterone level that is not bound and is active in stimulating target cells.

biphosphonates. A class of nonhormonal medication that blocks the breakdown of bone and results in increased bone formation.

bone mineral density. The measure of the amount of calcium and other minerals present in bone.

bone resorption. A process in which the body removes old bone to make way for new bone that forms in its place. This normal process is called bone remodeling.

chromosomes. The structural element of the cell nucleus that carries the hereditary material (genes). Chromosomes are condensed strands of DNA.

cognition. Sometimes called cognitive function, this term refers to the functioning capacity of the brain with respect to memory, learning, and other features of mental performance.

contraindications. Reasons not to take a drug or a treatment; required by the FDA to be included in package labeling of prescription drugs.

coronary. Refers to the main arteries that supply blood to the heart, the coronary arteries.

corpus luteum. The structure in the ovary that produces progesterone. It is formed from the vacated ovarian follicle after the egg is released (ovulation).

cytoplasm. A cell's internal fluid component and its contents.

DHEA. See *dehydroepiandrosterone.*

dehydroepiandrosterone. A prehormone produced in the body that is converted into testosterone. DHEAS refers to its sulfated form.

dementia. The broad term used to describe general cognitive dysfunction leading to loss of memory and other brain functions.

designer androgen. Drugs that act as androgens on some tissues and as androgen blockers (antiandrogens) on others. They are also known as SARMs (selective androgen receptor modifiers).

designer estrogens. Drugs that act as estrogens on some tissues and as estrogen blockers (antiestrogens) on others. They are also known as SERMs (selective estrogen receptor modifiers).

dihydrotestosterone. DHT; a major conversion product of testosterone that is even more potent and stimulatory to the prostate gland.

DNA. Chemical component of a cell that carries genetic information. It makes up the chromosomes which carry the cell's genes.

DNA fingerprinting. A chemical analysis done in the laboratory to chart the genetic material (coded in nucleic acids) unique to each individual.

ectopic pregnancy. Abnormal implantation of a fertilized egg in a location outside of the uterus, usually in the Fallopian tube; it can be life threatening if not diagnosed and treated.

endocrinology. The study of the body's organs of internal secretion (glands) and their products (hormones). Clinical endocrinologists diagnose and treat endocrine disorders; research endocrinologists study glands and hormonal actions.

endometrium. The inner lining cells of the uterus that grow and recede each month in response to hormone stimulation.

erectile dysfunction. The inability to have or maintain an erection because of a circulatory problem in the penis.

erythrocytes. Red blood cells.

erythropoiesis. The body's normal process of constantly synthesizing new red blood cells.

estradiol. The body's main estrogenic hormone produced by the ovary; it is also a conversion product of testosterone metabolism in both men and women.

estrogen receptor. The cellular element found in target cells (the uterus, for example) that binds to estrogen so that the combined estrogen and receptor complex can allow the hormone to act.

eugonadal. The term meaning that an individual is in a normal state of gonadal (ovary or testis) function.

exogenous hormones. Hormones not produced within the body but taken as a medication orally or by some other means of delivery.

fallopian tube. The convoluted tube that carries the egg from the surface of the ovary to the uterus. Meeting of egg and sperm takes place in its upper portion, near the ovary.

FDA. The United States Food and Drug Administration. This is the U.S. federal government agency that approves new drugs and monitors drugs on the market.

follicular phase. The first half of a woman's menstrual cycle when the ovarian follicle is developing and the hormone being produced by the ovary is predominantly estrogen.

free testosterone. The portion of the total testosterone in the blood that is not bound to its carrier protein. This is most of the bioavailable testosterone.

gonad. The sex gland; ovary in the female, testis in the male (sometimes called the testicle).

gonadal ridge. The earliest appearance of a structure in an embryo of a few weeks age that will go on to become an ovary or testis depending on the genetic sex determined at fertilization.

growth hormone. A large protein hormone produced by the pituitary gland that stimulates growth in children and has other effects on the body's metabolism.

hematopoiesis. The body's normal process of constantly forming new blood cells.

hippocampus. An area of the brain involved in memory.

human chorionic gonadotropin. HCG; the hormone of pregnancy that is produced by the placenta and by the zygote even earlier; it is the basis for detecting pregnancy in pregnancy tests.

hyperplasia. Excessive growth of a tissue that can be the precursor to cancer.

hypertension. High blood pressure.

hypogonadal. Less than normal gonadal (ovary or testis) function. It usually refers to young men with testicular insufficiency.

hypothalamus. The region at the base of the brain that produces small hormones that stimulate the underlying pituitary gland.

in vitro fertilization. IVF; an assisted reproduction technique in which egg and sperm are placed together in the laboratory so that fertilization occurs outside the body.

isoflavones. A group of substances in some plants that are estrogenic.

Kegel vaginal contractions. A type of exercise to strengthen the sphincter that holds the urine in the bladder.

Kupperman index. A scale of subjective measures of a woman's menopausal symptoms.

L-dopa. L-3,4-dihydroxyphenylalanine; a drug used for the treatment of Parkinson's disease and other neurological disorders.

Leydig cells. The cells of the testis that produce testosterone.

libido. The interest in and urge to have sex.

luteal phase. The second half of a woman's menstrual cycle when the predominant hormone being produced by the ovary is progesterone.

luteinizing hormone. LH; a protein hormone produced by the pituitary gland that stimulates the ovary in several ways, including the trigger to ovulate.

mammography. Taking an X-ray picture, called a mammogram, of the breast.

medullary tubes. The inner part of the gonadal ridge that develops into the testis and houses the primordial stem cells that eventually become sperm.

melatonin. A brain hormone produced in high amounts at an early age that gradually declines with aging. It is believed to have a role in sleep.

meta-analysis. Statistical analysis of several similar clinical trials combined to increase the power of conclusions.

molecular biology. The study of biology at the molecular level, focusing on understanding elements within the cells themselves, such as genes and gene products.

MRI. Magnetic resonance imaging; a noninvasive method to analyze internal organs such as the brain.

myocardial infarct. A heart attack usually caused by a lack of oxygen because of narrowing of the arteries that bring blood to the heart muscle.

myoma. A fibroid that grows abnormally in the muscular wall of the uterus (the myometrium).

myomectomy. Surgical removal of uterine fibroids.

myotropic activity. The term describing the ability of androgens to stimulate muscle growth.

neurophysiology. The study of the physiology of the body's nerve system.

neuropsychological tests. A battery of tests to evaluate memory and other aspects of brain function.

node-positive, node-negative. Terms used to indicate whether a cancer has spread to the nearby lymph nodes.

nonovulatory cycle. A menstrual cycle during which an egg is not released.

nutritional supplements. Classification of products that do not claim
to cure disease that can be sold without FDA approval and do not
require a doctor's prescription.

observational study. A clinical study in which people who are already
receiving a treatment are followed to learn about the safety and effectiveness of one therapy as compared to another; a less than ideal
study design because there is no random selection process and
unknown, uncontrolled factors could be at play.

oogonia. The embryonic stem cells that eventually develop into an egg.

osteopenia. A condition of moderate loss of bone minerals.

osteoporosis. A condition of severe loss of bone mineral density that
can lead to fractures, especially of the hips and spine.

ovulation. The release of an egg from the ovary normally around the
14th day of the menstrual cycle; it can be induced by fertility drugs.

ovulatory cycle. A menstrual cycle during which an egg is successfully
released at about mid-cycle.

perimenopause. The few years just before menstrual periods stop completely due to menopause; intermittent symptoms of menopause
may occur during this period.

PETscan. Positron emission tomography; a noninvasive procedure
that can measure blood flow in the brain.

phytoestrogens. Estrogens derived from a plant source.

pituitary gland. The gland located at the base of the brain that releases
a number of protein hormones that control the function of other
glands in the body.

placebo. An inactive substance that looks the same as and is administered in the same way as a drug in a clinical trial.

primordial follicles. The first structure in the developing ovary that eventually gives rise to the mature follicles that release an egg each
month and produce female hormones.

progesterone. The female hormone that acts on the uterus to prepare
it each month for receiving a fertilized egg.

progestins. The group of progesteronelike hormones used in hormone
replacement therapy and other treatments.

prostate-specific antigen. PSA; a protein in the blood that can be detected
by a test to indicate the early presence of prostate cancer.

puberty. The time of life when the testis or ovary of an adolescent starts
to be activated and release its hormones; in females it is also called

the menarche because it is accompanied by the beginning of menstrual periods.

pulmonary embolism. A blood clot migrating to the lung from a vein in which blood clotting has occurred.

randomized clinical trial. A type of trial in which two types of treatment or no treatment are used to learn how the treatments affect groups of subjects; subjects are randomly assigned to one group or the other. This type of trial is considered more reliable than observational studies.

reductase, 5α. The enzyme responsible for converting testosterone into the more potent dihydrotestosterone.

regimen. A treatment plan that specifies the dosage, schedule, and duration of treatment.

SARM. Selective androgen receptor modifier; see *designer androgen.*

seminiferous tubules. The tightly packed, convoluted tubules that make up almost all of the bulk of the mature testis. Sperm production takes place within the tubules.

serotonin. A chemical messenger that transmits stimuli from one nerve cell to another in the brain (a neurotransmitter); believed to be associated with depression.

SERM. Selective estrogen receptor modifier; see *designer estrogen.*

sex determination. The establishment of genetic sex at fertilization, dependent on whether an X-chromosome-bearing sperm (female) or Y-chromosome-bearing sperm (male) fertilizes the egg.

sex differentiation. The gradual development of male or female sex organs and characteristics during the growth of the fetus.

sex hormone binding globulin. SHBG; the carrier protein in the blood that binds most of the testosterone in circulation, keeping it from exerting its androgenic activity.

sleep apnea. An occasional interruption of breathing during sleep which can cause sudden awakening.

sonogram. An ultrasound display of characteristics of internal organs, such as the thickness of the uterine lining.

spermatogonia. The primordial stem cells of the testis that will ultimate mature into sperm; present in the normal testis throughout life.

stacking. The practice of using several androgenic products at the same time; practiced by body builders with the expectation of getting increased muscle building.

stem cell. An early embryonic cell with the potential to become almost any kind of tissue if given the proper stimuli.

supine. Lying on one's back as opposed to standing upright.

suprapharmacological. A dose of a medication that is extremely high, well above a level considered within acceptable limits.

tamoxifen. A synthetic compound known as a designer estrogen or SERM; has an estrogen-blocking effect on breast tissue.

target cells. In endocrinology, the cells programmed to respond to a specific hormone because they possess receptors that can attach to that hormone.

testosterone. A hormone produced in the testes of men and the ovaries of women and in the adrenal glands of both sexes; its main role is to stimulate masculine characteristics in men; in women it appears to be mood elevating and heightens sexual desire (libido).

testosterone esters. Man-made molecules in which side chains of various lengths are added by chemists to the testosterone molecule to alter the way it is absorbed into the body.

thrombophlebitis. The acute condition of having a large clot lodged in a vein that causes irritation and pain.

thrombosis. The formation of a blood clot, usually in a large vein (venous thrombosis).

transdermal delivery system. A method for delivering drugs to the body through the skin into the general circulation.

triglycerides. A lipid component of the blood serum ssociated with cholesterol values as part of the lipid profile; elevated trigyceride levels are risk factors for heart disease.

tubal-uterine junction. The entry point of the fallopian tube into the wall of the upper portion of the uterus.

U.S. Pharmacopoeia. USP; a nongovernmental organization that establishes standards to ensure the quality of medicines; officially recognized by U.S. law.

vasomotor lability. A condition that causes hot flashes; blood vessels of the skin become unstable (vasomotor instability) and dilate to allow a large amount of blood to flow through, causing flushing, heat, perspiration, and clamminess.

urinary incontinence. Sudden and uncontrolled loss of urine from the bladder.

zygote. The earliest stages of development after an egg is fertilized and before it implants into the uterine lining (the endometrium) and becomes an embryo.

• • • References

Chapter 1

Adashi EY. The ovarian follicular apparatus. In: Reproductive Endocrinology, Surgery and Technology, vol. 1, 46–70. Adashi EY, Rock J, Rosenwaks Z (Eds.). Lippincott-Raven, Philadelphia, 1996.

Coutinho E, Segal SJ. Is Menstruation Obsolete? Oxford University Press, New York, 1999.

Himelstein-Braw R, Byshou AG, Peters H, Faber M. Follicular atresia in the infant human ovary. J Reprod Fertil 46: 55, 1976.

Hodgen GD. The dormant ovarian follicle. Fertil Steril 38: 281–289, 1982.

Ichinoe K, Segal SJ, Mastroianni L Jr, Eds. Preservation of Tubo-Ovarian Function in Gynecologic Benign and Malignant Diseases. Serono Symposia Publications. Raven Press, New York, 1988.

Palumbo A, Yeh J. Apoptosis as a basic mechanism in the human cycle: Follicular atresia and luteal regression. J Soc Gynecol Invest 2: 565–573, 1995.

Peters H. Intrauterine gonadal development. Fertil Steril 27: 493–500, 1976.

Speroff L, Glass RH, Kase NJ. Clinical Gynecologic Endocrinology and Infertility. Williams & Wilkins, Baltimore, MD, 2000.

Yeh J, Adashi E. The ovarian life cycle. In: Reproductive Endocrinology, Physiology, Pathology and Clinical Management, 4th Ed., Yen SSC, Jaffe RB, Barbieri RL (Eds.). WB Saunders, Philadelphia, 1999, pp. 153–190.

Yen SSC. The human menstrual cycle: Neuroendocrine regulation. In: Reproductive Endocrinology, Physiology, Pathology and Clinical Management, 4th ed., Yen SSC, Jaffe RB, Barbieri RL (Eds.). WB Saunders, Philadelphia, 1999, pp. 191–217.

Witschi E. Migration of the germ cells in human ovaries. Proc Soc Biol 158: 417–425, 1963.

Chapter 2

Barlow DH, Cardozo LD, Francis RM, et al. Urogenital aging and its effect on sexual health in older British women. Br J Obstet Gynaecol 104: 87–95, 1997.

Bhatig V, Tchou DCH. Pelvic floor musculature exercise in treatment of anatomical stress incontinence. Physical Ther 68: 652–655, 1988.

Brown JS, Vittinghoff E, Kanaga AM, et al. Urinary tract infections in postmenopausal women: Effect of hormone therapy and risk factors. Obstet Gynecol 98: 1045–1054, 2001.

Dennerstein L, Dudley EC, Hopper JL, Guthrie JL, Burger HG. A prospective population-based study of menopausal symptoms. Obstet Gynecol 96: 351–359, 2000.

Fantly JA, Bump RC, Robinson D, McClish DK, Wyman JT. Efficacy of estrogen supplementation in the treatment of urinary incontinence. The continence program for Women's Research Group. Obstet Gynecol 88: 745–753, 1996.

Greendale GA, Reboussin BA, Hogan P, et al. Symptom relief and side effects of postmenopausal hormones: Results from the Postmenopausal Estrogen/Progestin Interventions Trial. Obstet Gynecol 92: 982–989, 1998.

Guthrie J, et al. Hot flushes, menstrual states and hormone levels in a population-based sample of midlife women. Obstet Gynecol 88: 437–442, 1996.

Subak LL, Quesenberry CP Jr, Posner SF, Cattolica E, Doghikian K. The effect of behavioral therapy on urinary incontinence: A randomized controlled trial. Obstet Gynecol 100: 72–78, 2002.

Chapter 3

Archer DF, First K, Tepping D, et al. A randomized comparison of continuous transdermal deliver of estradiol-norethindrone acetate and estradiol alone for menopause. CombiPatch Study Group. Obstet Gynecol 94: 498–503, 1999.

Archer DF, Pichar JH, Bottiglioni F. Bleeding patterns in post menopausal women taking continuous combined or sequential regimens of conjugated estrogens with medroxyprogesterone acetate. Obstet Gynecol 83: 686–691, 1994.

Bachman GA. The clinical platform for the 17 beta-estradiol vaginal releasing ring. Am J Obstet Gynecol 178: S251–S254, 1998.

Hargrove JT, Maxson WS, Wentz AC, Burnett LS. Menopausal hormone replacement therapy with continuous daily oral micronized estradiol and progesterone. Obstet Gynecol 73: 606, 1989.

Makinen J, Pitkanen VA, Salmi TA, et al. Transdermal estrogen for female stress urinary incontinence in post menopause. Maturitas 22: 1233–1238, 1995.

Raz R, Stam WE. A controlled trial of intravaginal estrial in postmenopausal women with recurrent urinary tract infections. N Engl J Med 329: 753, 1993.

Udoff L, Langenberg P, Adashi E. Combined continuous hormone replacement therapy: A critical review. Obstet Gynecol 86: 306–310, 1995.

Weinstein L, Beutra C, Gallagher JC. Evaluation of a continuous low-dose regimen of estrogen-progesterone for treatment of the menopausal patient. Am J Obstet Gynecol 162: 1534–1539, 1990.

Chapter 4

Antonijevec IA, Stolla GK, Steiger A, Modulation of the sleep electroencephalopgram by estrogen replacement in postmenopausal women. Am J Obstet Gynecol 182: 277–281, 2000.

Barlow DH, Cardozo LP, Francis RM, et al. Urogenital aging and its effects on sexual health in older British women. Br J Obstet Gynecol 104: 82–87, 1997.

Barrett-Connor E, Young R, Notelovitz M, Sullivan J, Witta B, Yang HM, et al. A two year double-blind comparison of estrogen-androgen and conjugated estrogen in surgically postmenopausal women. Effects on bone mineral density, symptoms and lipid profiles. J Reprod Med 44: 1012–1020, 1999.

Bravo J, Gunther P, Roy PM, Payette H, Gaulin P, Harvey M, et al. Impact of a 12-month exercise program on the physician and psychological health of osteopenic women. J Am Geriatr Soc 44: 756–762, 1996.

Cardozo LD, Kelleher CJ. Sex hormones, the menopause and urinary problems. Gynecol Endocrinol 9: 75–80, 1995.

Casper RF, Dodin S, Reid RL. The effect of 20 µg ethinyl estradiol/1 mg norethindrone acetate, a low dose oral contraceptive on vaginal bleeding patterns, hot flashes and quality of life in symptomatic perimenopausal women. Menopause 4: 139–143, 1997.

Cauley JH, Seeley DF, Ettinger B, Black D, Cummings GK, for the Study of Osteoporotic Fractures Research Group. Estrogen replacement therapy and fractures in older women. Ann Int Med 122: 9–16, 1995.

Collins A, Landgren BM. Psychosocial factors associated with the use of hormone replacement therapy in a longitudinal followup of Swedish women. Maturitas 28: 1–7, 1997.

Cummings SR, Browner WS, Bauer D, Stone K, Ensrud K, Jamal S, et al. Endogenous hormones and the risk of hip and vertebral fractures among older women. Study of Osteoporotic Fractures Research Group. N Engl J Med 339: 733–778, 1998.

Dawson-Hughes B, Harris SS, Krall EA, Dallal GE. Effect of calcium and vitamin D supplementation on bone density in men and women 65 years of age or older. N Engl J Med 337: 670–676, 1997.

Derman JJ, Dawood MY, Stone S. Quality of life during sequential hormone replacement therapy. A placebo-controlled study. Int J Fertil 40: 73–77, 1995.

Dinnerstein L, Dudley EC, Hopper JL, Guthrie JC, Burgett G. Population-based study of post-menopausal symptoms. Obstet Gynecol 96: 351–356, 2000.

Eastrell K. Treatment of osteoporosis. N Engl J Med 338: 736–746, 1998.

Fantl JA, Bump RC, Robinson D, Wyman JF. Efficiency of estrogen supplementation in the treatment of urinary incontinence. The Continua Program for Women Research Group. Obstet Gynecol 88: 745–751, 1996.

Greendale GA, Espeland M, Slone S, Marcus R, Barrett-Conner E. For the PEPI Safety followup Study (PSFS) Investigators. Bone mass response to discontinuation of long term hormone replacement therapy: Results from the Postmenopausal Estrogen/ Progestin Interventions (PEPI) Safety Followup Study. Arch Intern Med 62: 665–672, 2002.

Greendale GA, Reboussin BA, Hogan P, et al. Symptom relief and side effects of postmenopausal hormones: results from the postmenopausal estrogen/progestin interventional trial. Obstet Gynecol 92: 982–989, 1998.

Hays J, Ockene JK, Brunner RL, Kotchen JM, Manson JE, Patterson RE, Aragaki AK, Shumakre SA, Brzyski RG, LaCroix AZ, Granek IA, Valanis BG, for the Women's Health Initiative Investigators: Effects of Estrogen plus Progestin on Health Related Quality of Life. New Engl J Med 348(19), 2003.

Hlatky MA, Boothroyd B, Vittinghoff E, Sharp P, Whooley M. Quality-of-life and depressive symptoms in postmenopausal women after receiving hormone therapy. JAMA 287: 591–597, 2002.

Isaacs AJ, Brotten AR, McPherson K. Utilization of hormone replacement therapy by women doctors. Br Med J 311: 1139–1145, 1995.

Keefe DL, Watson K, Naftolin F. Hormone replacement therapy may alleviate sleep apnea in menopausal women: A pilot study. Menopause 6: 10–19, 1999.

Kolata G. Hormone Therapy, Already Found to Have Risks, Is Now Said to Lack Benefits. New York Times, March 18, 2003, p. A30.

Le Blanc ES, Janowsky J, Chan BK, Nelson HD. Hormone replacement therapy and cognition: systematic review and meta-analysis. JAMA 285: 1489–1499, 2001.

Lindsay R, Watts NB, Shoupe D. Current approaches to osteoporosis prevention. Am J Managed Care 4: 564–56-63, 1998.

Manson TE, Morton KA. Clinical practice. Post menopausal hormone replacement therapy. N Engl J Med 345: 34–39, 2001.

Oldenhave A, Jaszmann LJB, Haspels AA, Everaard W. Impact of climacteric on well-being: A survey based on 5213 women 39–60 years old. Am J Obstet Gynecol 168: 772–778, 1993.

Schneider DL, Barrett-Connor EC, Morton DJ. Timing of postmenopausal estrogen for optimal bone mineral density. JAMA 277: 543–547, 1997.

Shaver J, Giblin F, Lentz M, Lee K. Sleep patterns and stability in perimenopausal women. Sleep 11: 556–562, 1998.

Shiff I, Regestein G, Tulchinsky D, Ryan K. Effects of estrogen on sleep and psychological state. JAMA 242; 2405–2409, 1979.

Torgerson DT, Bell-Syer SE. Hormone replacement therapy and prevention of non-vertebral fractures: a meta analysis of randomized trials. JAMA 285: 2891–2897, 2001.

Tosteson AN, Gabriel SE, Kneeland TS, et al. Has the state of hypogonadal women in need of hormone replacement therapy and quality of life been improved? J Women's Health Gender Based Med 9: 119–124, 2000.

Utian WH, Boggs PP. The North American Menoapuse Society. 1998 Menopause Survey, Part 1: Postmenopausal women's perceptions about menopause and midlife. Menopause 122: 128–133, 1999.

Villareal DR, Binder FF, Williams DB, et al. Bone mineral density response to estrogen replacement in frail elderly women. JAMA 7: 815–820, 2001.

Watts NB, Notelovitz M, Timmons MC, Addison WA, Wiita B, Downey LJ. Comparison of oral estrogens and estrogens plus androgen on bone mineral density, menopausal symptoms and lipid-lipoprotein profiles in surgical menopause. Obstet Gynecol 85: 529–537, 1995.

Wimalawansa ST. Prevention and treatment of osteoporosis. Efficacy of combination hormone replacement therapy without antiresorptive agents. J Clin Densitom 3: 187–200, 2000.

Chapter 5

Angerer P, Stord S, Kothney W, et al. Effect of oral post menopausal hormone replacement on progression of atherosclerosis: a randomized controlled trial. Arterioschler Thromb Vas Biol 21: 202–208, 2001.

Archer DF, Dorin M, Lewis V, Schneider DL, Pickar JH. Effects of lower doses of conjugated equine estrogens and medroxyprogesterone acetate on endometrial bleeding. Fertil Steril 75: 1080–1087, 2001

Barrett-Connor E, Grady D, Sashegyi A, et al., for the MORE Investigators (Multiple Outcomes of Raloxifene Evaluation). Raloxifene and cardiovascular events in osteoporotic postmenopausal women: four-year results from the MORE (Multiple Outcomes of Raloxifene Evaluation) randomized trial. JAMA 287: 847–857, 2002.

Barrett-Connor E, Slone S, Greendale G, et al. The Postmenopausal Estrogen/Progestin Interventions Study: primary outcomes in adherent women. Maturitas 27: 261–274, 1997.

Cauley JA, Norton L, Lippman ME, et al. Continued breast cancer risk reduction in postmenopausal women treated with raloxifene: 4-year results from the MORE trial. Multiple outcomes of raloxifene evaluation. Breast Cancer Res Treat 65: 125–134, 2001.

Chlebowski RT, Hendrix SL, Langer RD, et al. Influence of estrogen and progestin on breast cancer and mammography in healthy postmenopausal women. JAMA 289: 3243–3253, 2003.

Collaborative Group on Human Factors in Breast Cancer and Hormone Replacement Therapy. Collaborative reanalysis of data from 51 epidemiologic studies of 52,705 women with breast cancer and 18,841 women without breast cancer. Lancet 350: 1047–1059, 1997.

Davidson M, Make KC, Mark P, et al. Effects of continuous estrogen and estrogen-progestin replacement regimens in cardiovascular risk markers in postmenopausal women. Arch Intern Med 160: 3315–3321, 2000.

Delmas PD, Ensrud KE, Adachi JD, et al., for the Multiple Outcomes of Raloxifene Evaluation Investigators. Efficacy of raloxifene on vertebral fracture risk reduction in postmenopausal women with osteoporosis: four-year results from a randomized clinical trial. J Clin Endocrinol Metab 87: 3609–3617, 2002.

Goldstein F, Newcomb PA, Stampler MJ. Postmenopausal hormone therapy and the risk of colorectal cancer: A review and meta-analysis. Am J Med 106: 574–582, 1999.

Grady D, Herrington D, Bittner V, et al., for the HERS Research Group. Cardiovascular disease outcomes during 6.8 years of hormone therapy: Heart and Estrogen/Progestin Replacement Study follow-up (HERS II). JAMA 288: 49–57, 2002.

Greendale GA, Espeland M, Slone S, Marcus R, Barrett-Connor E, for the PEPI Safety Follow-up Study (PSFS) Investigators. Bone mass response to discontinuation of long-term hormone replacement therapy: results from the Postmenopausal Estrogen/Progestin Interventions (PEPI) safety follow-up study. Arch Intern Med 162: 665–672, 2002.

Greendale GA, Wells B, Marcus R, Barrett-Connor E, for the Postmenopausal Estrogen/Progestin Interventions trial investigators. How many women lose bone mineral density while taking hormone replacement therapy? Results from the Postmenopausal Estrogen/Progestin Interventions trial. Arch Intern Med 160: 3065–3071, 2000.

Grimes DA and Lobo RA: Perspectives on the Women's Health Initiative Trial of Hormone Replacement Therapy. Obstet Gynecol 100: 1344–1353, 2002.

Grodstein F, Manson JF, Colditz GA, et al. A prospective observational study of postmenopausal hormone therapy and primary prevention of cardiovascular disease. Ann Intern Med 133: 93–97, 2000.

Grodstein F, Stampfer MJ, Colditz GA, et al. Postmenopausal hormone therapy and mortality. N Engl J Med 336: 1769–1775, 1997.

Grodstein F, Stampfer MJ, Manson JE, et al. Postmenopausal estrogen and progestin use and the risk of cardiovascular disease. N Engl J Med 335: 453–461, 1996.

Hechberg SK, Kaplan RC, Weiss NS, et al. Risk of recurrent coronary artery disease in relation to use and recent initiation of post menopausal hormone therapy. Arch Intern Med 161: 1709–1715, 2001.

Herrington DM, Howard TD, Hawkins GA, et al. Estrogen receptor polymorphisms and effects on estrogen replacement on high density lipoprotein cholesterol in women with coronary disease. N Engl J Med 346: 967–974, 2002.

Herrington DM, Reboussin DM, Brosnihan B, et al. Effects of estrogen replacement on the progression of coronary artery atherosclerosis. N Engl J Med 343: 522–529, 2001.

Herrington DM, Vittinghoff E, Lin F, et al., for the HERS Study Group. Statin therapy, cardiovascular events, and total mortality in the Heart and Estrogen/Progestin Replacement Study (HERS). Circulation 105: 2962–2967, 2002.

Hlatky MA, Boothroyd D, Vittinghoff E, Sharp P, Whooley MA, for the Heart and Estrogen/Progestin Replacement Study (HERS) Research Group. Quality-of-life and depressive symptoms in postmenopausal women after receiving hormone therapy: Results from the Heart and Estrogen/ Progestin Replacement Study (HERS) trial. JAMA 287: 591–597, 2002.

Hodis HN, Mack WJ, Lobo RA, et al, for Estrogen in the Prevention of Atherosclerosis Trial Research Group. Estrogen in the prevention of atherosclerosis: a randomized, double-blind, placebo-controlled trial. Ann Intern Med 135: 939–953, 2001.

Hsia J, Simon JA, Lin F, et al. Peripheral arterial disease in randomized trial of estrogen with progestin in women with coronary heart disease: the Heart and Estrogen/Progestin Replacement Study. Circulation 102: 2228–2232, 2000.

Huang M-H, Schocken M, Block G, et al. Variation in nutrient intakes by ethnicity: Results from the Study of Women's Health Across the Nation (SWAN). Menopause 9: 309–319, 2002.

Hulley S, Furberg C, Barrett-Connor E, et al., for the HERS Research Group. Noncardiovascular disease outcomes during 6.8 years of hormone therapy: Heart and Estrogen/Progestin Replacement Study follow-up (HERS II). JAMA 288: 58–66, 2002.

Hulley S, Grady D, Bush T, et al., for the Heart and Estrogen/progestin Replacement Study (HERS) Research Group. Randomized trial of estrogen plus progestin for secondary prevention of coronary heart disease in postmenopausal women. JAMA 280: 605–613, 1998.

Lindsay R, Gallagher JC, Kleerekoper M, Pickar JH. Effect of lower doses of conjugated equine estrogens with and without medroxyprogesterone acetate on bone in early postmenopausal women. JAMA 287: 2668–2676, 2002.

Lobo RA, Bush T, Carr BR, Pickar JH. Effects of lower doses of conjugated equine estrogens and medroxyprogesterone acetate on plasma lipids and lipoproteins, coagulation factors, and carbohydrate metabolism. Fertil Steril 76: 13–24, 2001.

Mandel J, Church T, Bend J, et al. The effect of fecal occult blood screening on the incidence of colorectal cancer. N Engl J Med 343: 1603–1607, 2000.

Mendelsohn ME, Karas RH. The time has come to stop letting the HERS tale wag the dogma. Circulation 104: 2256–2259, 2001.

Mosca L, Collins P, Harrington DM, et al. Hormone replacement therapy and cardiovascular disease: A statement for health care professionals from the American Heart Association. Circulation 104: 499–504, 2001.

Ornish D, Scherwitz LW, Billings JH, Gould L, Merrett T, et al. Intensive life style changes for reversal of coronal heart disease. JAMA 280: 2001–2007, 1998.

Persson I, Weiderpass E, Bergstrom R, Schairer C. Risks of breast and endometrial cancer after estrogen and estrogen-progestin replacement. Cancer Causes Control 10: 253–260, 1999.

Pickar JH, Yeh I, Wheeler JE, Cunnane MF, Speroff L. Endometrial effects of lower doses of conjugated equine estrogens and medroxyprogesterone acetate. Fertil Steril 76: 25–31, 2001.

Program on breast cancer and envionmental risk factors in New York State, Cornell University, Ithaca, New York, 2002.

Reiss E, Holnbrob K, Young JB, et al. Estrogen is associated with improved survival in aging woman with congestive heart failure. J Am Coll Cardiol 365: 24–29, 2000.

Ross RK, Paganini-Hill A, Wan PC, Pike MC. Effect of hormone replacement therapy on breast cancer risk: estrogen vs. estrogen plus progestin. J Natl Cancer Inst 92: 328–332, 2000.

Schairer C, Lubin J, Troisi R, Sturgen S, Brinton L, Hoover R. Menopausal estrogen and estrogen-progestin replacement therapy and breast cancer risk. JAMA 283: 485–491, 2000.

Sheele F, Burger CW, Kenemans P. Postmenopausal hormone replacement in the woman with a reproductive risk factor for breast cancer. Maturitas 33: 191–196, 1999.

Simon JA, Hsia J, Cauley JA, et al. Postmenopausal hormone therapy and risk of stroke: the Heart and Estrogen-progestin Replacement Study (HERS). Circulation 103: 638–642, 2001.

Speroff L. Postmenopausal hormone therapy and the risk of breast cancer. Maturitas 32: 123–129, 1999.

Utian WH, Shoupe D, Bachmann G, Pinkerton JV, Pickar JH. Relief of vasomotor symptoms and vaginal atrophy with lower doses of conjugated equine estrogens and medroxyprogesterone acetate. Fertil Steril 75: 1065–1079, 2001.

Viscoli CM, Brass LM, Kernan WN, Sarrel PM, Suissa S, Horwitz RI. A clinical trial of estrogen-replacement therapy after ischemic stroke. N Engl J Med 345: 1243–1249, 2001

Wassertheil-Smoller S, Hendrix S, Limacher M, et al. Effects of estrogen plus progestin on stroke in post-menopausal women. JAMA 289: 2673–2684, 2003.

Woolf S. The best screening test for colorectal cancer: A personal choice. N Engl J Med 343: 1641–1643, 2000.

Writing Group for the PEPI trial. Effects of hormone therapy on bone mineral density: Results from the Postmenopausal Estrogen/Progestin Interventions (PEPI) trial. JAMA 276: 1389–1396, 1996.

Writing Group for the Women's Health Initiative Investigators. Risks and benefits of estrogen plus progestin in healthy postmenopausal women: Principal results from the Women's Health Initiative randomized controlled trial. JAMA 288: 321–333, 2002.

Chapter 6

Anderson E, Hamberger S, Lia SJ, Rebar RW. Characteristics of postmenopausal women seeking assistance. Am J Obstet Gynecol 156: 428–433, 1987.

Ballinger CA. Psychiatric morbidity and the menopause: Screening of a general population sample. Br Med J 3: 344–346, 1975.

Coope T. Is oestrogen therapy effective in the treatment of menopausal depression? J R Coll Gen Pract 31: 134–140, 1981.

Hallstrom T, Samuelsson S. Mental health in the climacteric: The longitudinal study of women in gathenburg. Acta Obstet Gynecol Scand 130: 13–18, 1985.

Henderson VW, Paganini-Hill. Estrogen and Alzheimer's disease. J SOGC S21–S28–S31, 1997.

Henderson V, Watt L, Buckwalter JG. Cognitive skills associated with estrogen replacement in women with Alzheimer's disease. Psychoneuroendocrinology 21: 421–430, 1996.

Hogervost E, Williams T, Burger , Riedel W, Jolles J. The nature of the effect of female gonadal hormone replacement therapy on cognitive function in post menopausal women: a meta analysis. Neuroscience 101: 485–512, 2000.

Jover T, Tanaka H, Calderone A, et al. Estrogen protects against global ischemia-induced neuronal death and prevents activation of apoptotic signaling cascade in the hippocampal CA1. J Neuro 22(6): 2115–2124, 2002.

Kawas C, et al. A prospective study of estrogen replacement therapy and the risk of developing Alzheimer's disease. The Baltimore Longitudinal Study of Aging. Nuerology 48: 1517–1521, 1997.

Knopman D, Boland G, Mosley T, et al. Cardiovascular risk factors and cognitive decline in middle aged adults. Neurology 56: 42–48, 2001.

LeBlanc ES, Janowsky J, Chan BK, Nelson HD. Hormone replacement therapy and cognition: Systematic review and meta-analysis. J Am Med Assoc 285: 1489–1499, 2001.

MacKinlay SM, Brambilla DJ, Pasner JA. The normal menstrual transition. Maturitas 14: 103–105, 1992.

Mortola JF. Estrogens and mood. J SOGC S1–S6, 1997.

Rapp S, Espeland M, Shumaker S, et al. Effect of estrogen plus progestin on global cognitive function in postmenopausal women. JAMA 289: 2663–2672, 2003.

Rowe JW, Kahn R. Successful aging. Random House, New York. 1998.

Schneider LS, Small GW, Hamilton SH, et al. Estrogen replacement and response to fluoxetine in a multicenter geriatric depression trial. Fluoexitine Collaborative Study Group. Am J Geriatric Psychiatry 5: 97–106, 1997.

Sherwin BB, Carlson LE. Estrogen and memory in women. J SOGC S7–S13, 1997.

Sherwin BB, Gelfand MM. Sex steroids and effect on surgical menopause: A double blind crossover study. Psychoneuroendocrinology 10: 325–335, 1985.

Shumaker S, Legault C, Rapp S. Estrogen plus progestin and the incidence of dementia and mild cognitive impairment in postmenopausal women. JAMA 289: 2651–2661, 2003.

Simpkins JW, Green PS, Gribley KE, Shi J. Estrogens and memory protection. J SOGC S14–S20, 1997.

Soares CN, Almeida OP, Jaffe H, Cohen LS. Efficacy of estradiol for the treatment of depressive disorders in perimenopausal women: a double-blind randomized, placebo controlled trial. Arch Gen Psych 58: 529–535, 2001.

Tang MX, Jacobs D, Stern Y, et al. Effect of oestrogen during menopause on risk and age of onset of Alzheimer's disease. Lancet 348: 429–432, 1996.

Valdereschi M, et al. Estrogen replacement therapy and Alzheimer's disease in the Italian longitudinal study on aging. Neurology 50: 996–1002, 1998.

Zandi PP, et al. Hormone replacement therapy and incidence of Alzheimer's disease in older women. JAMA 288: 2123–2129, 2002.

Chapter 7

American Society for Reproductive Medicine. 2002 Guidelines for Gamete and Embryo donation. Fertil and Steril 77 (suppl. 6): 1S-18S, 2002.

Benadiva CA, Kligman I, Munne S. Aneuploidy 16 in human embryos increases significantly with maternal age. Fertil Steril 66: 248–255, 1996.

Cohen J, Scott R, Schimmel T, Levron J, Willadsen S. Birth of infant after transfer of anucleate donor oocyte cytoplasm into recipient eggs. Lancet 350: 186–187, 1997.

Dohle GR, Halley DJ, Van Hemel JO, van Den Ouwel AM, Pierers MH, Webers RF, Govaerts LC. Genetic risk factors in infertile men with severe oligozoospermia and azoospermia. Hum Reprod 17: 13–26, 2002.

Ethics Committee of the American Society for Reproductive Medicine. Financial incentives in recruitment of oocyte donors. Fertil Steril 74: 216–220, 2000.

Hawes SM, Sapienza C, Latham KE. Ooplasmic donation in humans: The potential for epigenic modifications. Hum Reprod 17: 850–852, 2002.

Mastroianni L Jr, Biggers J (Eds.). Fertilization and Embryonic Development In Vitro. Plenum Press, New York, 1981.

Mastroianni L Jr, Paulsen CA (Eds). Aging, Reproduction, and the Climacteric. Plenum Press, New York, 1986.

Menken J, Trussell J, Larsen U. Age and infertility. Science 233: 1389–1394, 1986.

Munne S, Cohen J, Sable D. Preimplantation genetic diagnosis for advanced maternal age and other indications. Fertil Ster 78: 234–236, 2002.

Sauer MV. Pregnancy after age 50: Application of oocyte donation to women after natural menopause. Lancet 341: 321–323, 1993.

Sauer MV, Paulson RJ, and Lobo, RA. A preliminary report on oocyte donation extending reproductive potential to women over 40. N Engl J Med J Med 323: 1157–1160, 1990.

Smith KE, Buyalos RP. The profound impact of patient age on pregnancy outcome after early detection of fetal cardiac activity. Fertil Steril 65: 35–40, 1996.

Society for Assisted Reproductive Technology. American Society for Reproductive Medicine. Assisted Reproductive Technology in the United States and Canada: 1998 Results from the American Society for Reproductive Medicine/Society for Assisted Reproductive Technology Registry. Fertil Steril 77: 18–30, 2002.

Taffe J, Dennerstein L. Time to the final menstrual period. Fertil Steril 78: 397–403, 2002.

Tarin JJ, Handyside AH. Embryo biopsy strategies for preimplantation diagnosis. Fertil Steril 59: 943–952, 1993.

Tureck RW, Garcia C-R, Blasco L, Mastroianni L. Perioperative complication arising after transvaginal oocyte retrieval. Obstet Gynecol 81: 590–593, 1993.

Van Steirteghem A, Joris H, Liu J, Nahy Z, Tournaye H, Leibaers I, Devroey P. Assisted fertilization by subzonal insemination and intracytoplasmic sperm injection. In Gamete and Embryo Quality, Mastroianni L, Coelingh Bennick H JT, Suzuki S, Vemer HHM (Eds.). Carnforth, UK: Parthenon, 1993, pp. 117–124.

Chapter 8

Eisenberg DM, Davis RB, Ettner SL, Appel S, Wilkey S, Van Rompay M, et al. Trends in alternative medicine use in the United States 1990–1997. Results of a follow-up survey. JAMA 280: 1569–1575, 1998.

Food and Drug Administration. Risk of drug interactions with St. John's Wort. JAMA 283–288: 1679, 2000.

Fugh-Berman A. Herb-drug interactions. Lancet 355: 134–138, 2000.

Gas MS. Taylor MB. Alternatives for women through menopause. Am J Obstet Gynecol 185(2) (suppl): S47–S56, 2001.

GlaxoSmithKline. Remifin Menopause product brochure. London UK, 2001.

Hirata JD, Swiersz LM, Zell BS, Small R, Ettinger B. Does dong quai have estrogenic effects in postmenopausal women? A double-blind, placebo controlled trial. Fertil Steril 68: 961–986, 1997.

Kass-Annese B. Alternative therapies for menopause. Am J Obstet Gynecol 43: 162–183, 2000.

Ko RJ. Adulterants in Asian patent medicines. N Engl J Med 339: 847–852, 1998.

North American Menopause Society. The role of isoflavones in menopausal health: Consensus opinion of the North American Menopause Society. Menopause 7: 215–229, 2000.

Physician's Desk Reference. Thompson Health Care, Montvale, NJ 2003.

Taylor M. Alternatives to conventional hormone replacement. Menopausal Med 6: 1–6, 1998.

Wiklund I, Mattsson L, Lindgren R, et al. Effects of a standardized ginsing extract on a double-blind placebo controlled trial. Int J Clin Pharm Res 19: 89–99, 1999.

Chapter 9

Albertazzi P, Pansini F, Bonaccorsi G, Zanotti L, Forini E, DeAloysio D. The effect of dietary soy supplementation on hot flushes. Obstet Gynecol 91: 6–11, 1998.

Anderson JW, Johnstone BM, Cook-Newell ME. Meta-analysis of the effects of soy protein intake on serum lipids. N Engl J Med 333: 276–282, 1995.

Baird DD, Umbach DM, Lansdell L, Hughes CL, Setchell KD, Weinberg CR, et al. Dietary intervention study to assess estrogenicity of dietary soy among postmenopausal women. J Clin Endocrinol Metab 80: 1685–1690, 1995.

Balk JL, Whiteside DA, Naus G, DeFerrari E, Roberts JM. A pilot study of the effects of phytoestrogen supplementation on postmenopausal endometrium. J Soc Gynecol Invest 9: 238–242, 2002.

Clarkson TB, Anthony MS, Williams JK, Honore EK, Cline M. The potential of soybean phytoestrogens for post menopausal hormone replacement therapy. Proc Soc Exp Biol Med 217: 365–368, 2002.

Duncan AM, Underhill KE, Xu X, Lavalleur J, Phipps WR, Kurzer MS. Modest hormonal effects of soy isoflavones in postmenopausal women. J Clin Endocrinol Metab 84: 3479–3484, 1999.

Glazier MG, Bowman MA. A review of the evidence for the use of phyto-estrogens as a replacement for traditional estrogen replacement therapy. Arch Intern Med 161: 1161–1172, 2001.

Han KK, Soares JM, Harder MA, Rodgirues de Lima G, Baraat F. Benefits of soy isoflavone therapeutic regimen on menopausal symptoms. Obstet Gynecol 99: 389–394, 2002.

Nestel PJ, Pomeroy S, Kay S, Komesaroff P, Behrsing J, Cameron JD, et al. Isoflavones from red clover improve systemic arterial compliance but not plasma lipids in menopausal women. J Clin Endocrinol Metab 84: 895–898, 1999.

North American Menopause Society. The role of isoflavones in menopausal health: Consensus opinion of the North American Menopause Society. Menopause 7: 215–229, 2000.

Pino AM, Calladares LE, Palma MA, Mancills AM, Yanez M, Albala C. Dietary isoflavones affect sex hormone binding globulin levels in postmenopausal women. J Clin Endocrinol Metab 85: 2797–2800, 2000.

Quella SK, Loprinzi CL, Barton DL, Knost JA, Sloan JA, LaVasseru BI, et al. Evaluation of soy phytoestrogens for the treatment of hot flashes in breast cancer survivors: A North Central Cancer Treatment Group Trial. J Clin Oncol 18: 1068–1074, 2000.

Simons LA, von Konigsmark M, Simons J, Celermajer DS. Phytoestrogens do not influence lipoprotein levels or endothelial function in healthy, postmenopausal women. Am J Cardiol 85: 1297–1301, 2000.

St. Germain A, Peterson CT, Robinson JG, Alekei DL. Isoflavone-rich or isoflavone-poor soy protein does not reduce menopausal symptoms during 24 weeks of treatment. Menopause 8: 17–26, 2001.

This P, De La Rochefordiere A, Clough K, Fourquet A, Magdelenat H. Phytoestrogens after breast cancer. Endocr Relat Cancer 8: 129–134, 2001.

Tikkanen MK, Wahala K, Ojala S, Vihrna V, Adlercreutz H. Effect of soybean phytoestrogen intake on low density lipoprotein oxidation resistance. Proc Natl Acad Sci USA 95: 3106–3110, 1998.

Upmalis DH, Lobo R, Bradley L, Warren M, Cone FL, Lamie CA. Vasomotor symptom relief by soy isoflavone extract tablets in postmenopausal women: A multicenter, double-blind, randomized, placebo controlled study. Menopause 7: 236–242, 2000.

Chapter 10

Artl W, Callies F, Allolio B. DHEA replacement in women with adrenal insufficiency—pharmacokinetics, bioconversion and clinical effects on well-being, sexuality and cognition. Endocr Res 26: 505–511, 2000.

Arlt W, Callies F, van Vlijmen JC, Koehler I, Reincke M, Bidlingmaier M, et al. Dehydroepiandrosterone replacement in women with adrenal insufficiency. N Engl J Med 341: 1013–1020, 1999.

Bachmann GA. The hypoandrogenic woman: pathophysiologic overview. Fertil Steril 77 (Suppl 4): S72–S76, 2002.

Bachman G, et al. Female androgen insufficiency: The Princeton consensus statement on definition, classification, and assessment. Fertil Steril 77: 660–665, 2002.

Bancroft J. Sexual effects of androgens in women: some theoretical considerations. Fertil Steril 77 (suppl. 4): S55–S59, 2002.

Braunstein GD. Androgen insufficiency in women: summary of critical issues. Fertil Steril 77 (suppl. 4): S94–S99, 2002.

Burger HG, Dudley EC, Cui J, Dennerstein L, Hopper JL. A prospective longitudinal study of serum testosterone dehydroepiandrosterone sulphate and sex hormone binding flobulin levels through the menopause transition. J Clin Endocrinol Metab 85: 2832–2938, 2000.

Celotto F, Melcangi RC, Negri-Cesi P, Poletti A. Testosterone metabolism in brain cells and membranes. J Steroid Biochem Mol Biol 40: 673–678, 1991.

Couzinet B, Meduri G, Lecce M, Young J, Brailly S, Loosfelt H, et al. The post menopausal ovary is not a major androgen producing gland. J Clin Endocinol Metab 86: 5060–5065, 2001.

Davis SR. Androgen replacement in women: A commentary. J Clin Endocrinol Metab 84: 1886–1891, 1999.

Davis SR. The therapeutic use of androgens in women. J Steroid Biochem Mol Biol 69: 177–184, 1999.

Davis SR. When to suspect androgen deficiency other than at menopause. Fertil Steril 77 (suppl. 4): S68–S71, 2002.

Davis SR, Burger HG. Androgens and the postmenopausal woman. J Clin Endocrinol Metab 81: 2759–2764, 1996.

Dennerstein L, Randolph J, Taffe J, Dudley E, Burger H. Hormones, mood, sexuality, and the menopausal transition. Fertil Steril 77 (suppl. 4): S42–S47, 2002.

Guay AT. Screening for androgen deficiency in women: methodological and interpretive issues. Fertil Steril 77, (suppl. 4): S83–S88, 2002.

Guzick DG, Hager K. Sex hormones and hysterectomies. N Engl J Med 343: 730–734, 2000.

Hickok LR, Toomey C, Speroff L. A comparison of esterified estrogen with and without methyltestosterone: Effects of endometrial histology and serum lipoproteins in postmenopausal women. Obstet Gynecol 82: 919–924, 1993.

Laughlin GA, Barrett-Connor E, Kritz-Silverstein D, Von Muhlen D. Hysterectomy, oophorectomy, and endogenous sex hormone levels in older women: The Rancho Bernardo Study. J Clin Endocrinol Metab 85: 645–651, 2000.

Leiblum S, Bachmann G, Kemmann E, Colburn DS, Swartzmann L. Vaginal atrophy in the postmenopausal woman: the importance of sexual activity and hormones. JAMA 249: 2195–2198, 1984.

Manson JE, Martin KA. Postmenopausal hormone replacement therapy. N Engl J Med 354: 34–40, 2001.

Miller KK, Sesmilo G, Schiller A, Schoenfeld D, Burton S, Klibanski A. Androgen deficiency in women with hypopituitarism. J Clin Endocrinol Metab 86: 561–567, 2001.

Mushayandebvu T, Castracane DV, Gimpel T, Adel T, Santoro N. Evidence for diminished midcycle ovarian androgen production in older reproductive aged women. Fertil Steril 65: 721–723, 1996.

Notelovitz M, Nanavati MS, Mazzeo M. Estradiol absorption from vaginal tablets in postmenopausal women. Obstet Gynecol 99: 556–562, 2002.

Rosen RC. Assessment of femal sexual dysfunction: review of validated methods. Fertil Steril 77 (suppl. 4): S89–S92, 2002.

Sherwin BB. Randomized clinical trials of combined estrogen-androgen preparations: Effects on sexual functioning. Fertil Steril 77 (suppl. 4): S49–S54, 2002.

Sherwin BB, Gelfand MM. The role of androgen in the maintenance of sexual functioning in oophorectomized women. Psychosom Med 49: 397–409, 1987.

Sherwin BN, Gelfand MM, Brender W. Androgen enhances sexual motivation in females. A perspective, cross over study of sex steroid administration in surgical menopause. Psychosom Med 47: 339–351, 1997.

Sherwin BB, Gelfand MM, Schucher R, Gabor J. Postmenopausal estrogen and androgen replacement and lipoprotein lipid concentrations. Am J Obstet Gynecol 156: 414–419, 1987.

Shifran JL, Braunstein GD, Simon JA, et al. Transdermal testosterone treatment in women with impaired sexual function after oophorectomy. N Engl J Med 343: 682–687, 2000.

Simon JA. Estrogen replacement therapy: Effects on the endogenous androgen milieu. Fertil Steril 77 (suppl. 4): S77–S82, 2002.

Simpson ER, Rubin G, Clyne C, Robertson K, O'Donnell L, Jones M, et al. The role of local estrogen biosynthesis in males and females. Trends Endocrinol Metab 11: 184–188, 2000.

Tuiten A, Laan E, Panhuysen G, Everaerd W, de Haan E, Koppeschaar H, et al. Discrepancies between genital responses and subjective sexual function during testosterone substitution in women with hypothalamic amenorrhea. Psychosom Med 58: 234–241, 1996.

Zumoff B, Strain GW, Miller LK, Rosner W. Twenty-four-hour mean plasma testosterone concentration declines with age in normal premenopausal women. J Clin Endocrinol Metab 80: 1429–1430, 1995.

Chapter 11

Baker VL, Draper M, Paul S, et al. Reproductive endocrine and endometrial effects of raloxifene hydrochloride, a selective estrogen receptor modulator, in women with regular menstrual cycles. J Clin Endocrin Metab 83: 6–13, 1998.

Boss SM, Huster WJ, Neild JA, et al. Effects of raloxifene hydrochloride on the endometrium of postmenopausal women. Am J Obstet Gynecol 177: 1458–1464, 1997.

Cummings SR, Eckert S, Krueger KA, Grady D, Powles RJ, Cauley JA, et al. The effect of raloxifene on risk of breast cancer in postmenopausal women: Results from the MORE Trial. J Am Med Assoc 281: 2189–2197, 1999.

Delmas PD, Bjarnason NH, Mitlak BH, et al. Effects of raloxifene on bone mineral density, serum cholesterol concentrations, and uterine endometrium in postmenopausal women. N Engl J Med 337: 1641–1647, 1997.

Draper MW, Flowers DE, Huster WJ, et al. A controlled trial of raloxifene (LY139481) HCI: impact on bone turnover and serum lipid profile in healthy postmenopausal women. J Bone Mineral Res 11: 835–842, 1996.

Gradishar WJ, Jordan VC. The clinical potential of new antiestrogens. J Clin Oncol 15: 480–489, 1997.

Hammer M, Christou S, Nathorgt-Boos J, Reed T, Garre K. A double-blind randomized trial comparing the effects of tibolone and continuous hormone replacement therapy in postmenopausal women with menopausal symptoms. Br J Obstet Gynecol 105: 904–909, 1998.

Heaney RP, Draper MW. Raloxifene and estrogen: Comparative bone-remodeling kinetics. J Clin Endocrinol Metab 82: 3425–3429, 1997.

Jordan VC. Tamoxifen: The herald of a new era of preventative therapeutics. J Natl Cancer Inst 89: 741–749, 1997.

Love RR, Barden HS, Mazess RB, Epstein S, Chappell RJ. Effects of tamoxifen on lumbar spine bone mineral density in postmenopausal women after 5 years. Arch Intern Med 154: 2585–2588, 1994.

Love RR, Mazess RB, Varden HS, et al. Effects of tamoxifen on bone mineral density in postmenopausal women with breast cancer. N Engl J Med 326: 852–856, 1992.

Lum SS, Wolterine EA, Fletcher WS, Pommier RF. Changes in serum estrogen levels in women during tamoxifen therapy. Am J Surg 173: 399–402, 1997.

Mitalk BH, Cohen FJ. In search of optimal long-term female hormone replacement: The potential of selective estrogen receptor modulators. Horm Res 48: 155–163, 1997.

Vandenberg G, Yen SSC. Effect of anti-estrogenic action of clomiphene during the menstrual cycle: Evidence for a change in feedback sensitivity. J Clin Endocrinol Metab 37: 356, 1973.

Walsh BW, Kuller LH, Wild RA, Sofia P, Farmer D, Lawrence JB, Shah AS, Anderson PW. Effects of raloxifene on serum lipids and coagulation factors in healthy postmenopausal women. JAMA 279: 1445–1451, 1998.

Chapter 12

Bremner WJ, Vitiello MV, Prinz RN. Loss of circadian rhythm in blood testosterone levels with aging in normal men. J Clin Endocrinol Metab 56: 1278–1281, 1983.

Cunningham A. (Ed.) Guinness Book of Records. Bantam Books, New York, 2002.

Davidson, JM, Chen JJ, Cerapo L, Gray, GD, Greenleaf, WJ, Catania JA. Hormonal changes and sexual function in aging men. J Clin Endocrinol Metab 47: 71–77, 1983.

Fawcett DW. The ultrastructure and functions of the Sertoli cell. In: Frontiers in Reproduction and Fertility Control, Greep RO (Ed.). MIT Press, Cambridge, 1977, pp. 353–377.

Gray A, Feldman HA, McKinlay JB, Longcope C. Age, disease, and changing sex hormone levels in middle-aged men: results of the Massachusetts Male Aging Study. J Clin Endocrinol Metab 73: 1016–1025, 1991.

Heller CG, Clermont Y. Spermatogenesis in man: An estimate of its duration. Science Vol. 140, No. 3563: 184–186, 1963.

Lamberts SWJ, van der Beld AW, van der Lely AJ. The endocrinology of aging. Science 278: 419–424, 1997.

Lipsett MB. Sertoli cell function. In: The Human Testis, Rosemberg E, and Paulsen CA (Eds.). Plenum Press, New York, 1973, pp. 407–437.

Segal SJ. The testis: Development, maturation and physiology. In: Human Reproduction and Sexual Behavior, Lloyd CW (Ed.). Lea and Febiger, Philadelphia, 1964, pp. 50–79.

Segal SJ. The physiology of human reproduction. Sci Am September 23: 29–40, 1974.

Segal SJ, Nelson WO. Initiation and maintenance of testicular function. In: Recent Progress in the Endocrinology of Reproduction, Lloyd CW (Ed.). Academic Press, New York, 1959, pp. 107–130.

Sparrow D, Bosse R, Rowe, JW. The influence of age and body build on gonadal function in men. J Clin Endocrinol Metab 51: 508–512, 1980.

Witschi E. Migration of the germ cells of human embryos from the yolk-sac to the primitive gonadal filds, Contributions to Embryology no. 209. Carnegie Institution, Washington, DC, 1948.

Yen SSC, Jaffe RB, Barbieri RL. Reproductive Endocrinology: Physiology, Pathophysiology, and Clinical Management, 4th ed. W.B. Saunders, Philadelphia, 1970.

Chapter 13

Clark, JH et al. Mechanism of action of steroid hormones. In: William's Textbook of Endocrinology, 8th ed., Wilson JD, Foster DW (Eds). W.B. Saunders, Philadelphia, 111–132, 1992.

Eik-Nes, KD. Leydig Cells, 142. In: The Androgens of the Testis, Eik-Nes, KD (Ed.). Marcel Decker, New York, 1970.

Vermeulin A. Androgens in the aging male. J Clin Endocrinol Metab 73: 221–224, 1991.

Wilson, JD. Hormones and hormone action. In: Harrison's Principles of Internal Medicine, 13th ed. Isselbacher, K et al. (Eds.). McGraw-Hill, New York, 486–499, 1998.

Yen SSC, Jaffe RB, Barbieri RL (Eds). Reproductive Endocrinology, Physiology, Pathology and Clinical Management, 4th ed., W.B. Saunders, Philadelhia, 1999.

Chapter 14

Barrett-Connor E, Khan KT, Yen SS. A prospective study of dehydroepiandrosterone sulfate, mortality, and cardiovascular disease. N Engl J Med 315: 1519–2244, 1986.

Crook D. Androgen therapy in the aging male: assessing the effect on heart disease. Aging Male 2: 151–156, 1999.

Davidson JM, Chen JJ, Crapo L et al. Hormonal changes and sexual function in aging men. J Clin Endocrinol Metab 57: 71–77, 1984.

Feldman, HA, Longcope, C, Derby CA, et al. Age trends in the level of serum testosterone and other hormones in middle-aged men: Longitudinal results from the Massachusetts male aging study. J Clin Endocrinol Metab 87: 589–598, 2002.

Garfinkel D. Laudon M, Nof D, Zisapel N. Improvmement of sleep quality in elderly people by controlled release of melatonin. Lancet 346: 541–544, 1995.

Hayes, FJ. Testosterone—fountain of youth or drug of abuse? J Clin Endocrinol Metab 85: 3020–3023, 2000.

Kalimi M, Regelson W (Eds.). The Biological Role of Dehydroepiandrosterone. Walter de Gruyter, New York, 1990.

Kasperk CH, Wegedal, GE, Farley, JR, Linkhart TA, Turner RT, Baylink DJ. Androgens directly stimulate proliferation of bone cells *in vitro*. Endocrinology 124: 1576–1578, 1989.

Kwan M, Greenleaf WJ, Mann J, et al. The nature of androgen action on male sexuality: A combined laboratory—self-report study of hypogonadal men. J Clin Endocrinol Metab 57: 557–562, 1984.

Lam PL, Jimenez M, Zhuang, TN, et al. A double-blind, placebo controlled, randomized clinical trial of transdermal dihydrotestosterone gel on

muscular strength, mobility, and quality of life in older men with
partial androgen deficiency. J Clin Endocrinol Metab 86: 4078–4088,
2001.

Maro R, Williams I, Ling S, et al. Dehydroepiandrosterone inhibits human
vascular smooth muscle cell proliferation independent of ARs and ERs.
J Clin Endocrinol Metab 87 176–1811, 2002.

Marsh JD, Lehmann MH, Ritchie RH, Gwathmey JK, Green GE, Schlingar
RJ. Androgen receptors mediate hypertrophy in cardiac myocytes.
Circulation, 98: 256–261, 1998.

Medical Post. Gel better than patch for applying testosterone. July 18, 2000,
vol. 36, no.26.

Medical Post. Male hormone supplements not bad for heart after all. April 21,
1998, vol. 34, no 15.

Medical Post. Men with chronic angina benefit from testosterone patch. July
18, 2000, vol. 36, no.26.

Medical Post. N.A. Menopause Society. Testosterone replacement therapy still
risky. Nov. 6, 2001, vol. 37, no. 37.

Medical Post. Testosterone helps build muscle mass. October 16, 2001,
vol. 37, no. 35.

Orentreich N, Brind JL, Vogelman JH, Andres R, Baldwin H. Long-term
longitudinal measurements of plasma dehydroepiandrosterone sulfate in
normal men. J Clin Endocrinol Metab 75: 1002–1004, 1992.

Schill W-B. Fertility and sexual life of men after their forties and in older age.
Asian J Androl Mar 3 (1): 1–7, 2001.

Sheffield Moore, M, Urban, RJ, Wolf, SE, et al. Short term oxandrolone
administration stimulates net muscle protein synthesis in young men.
J Clin Endocrinol Metab 84: 2705–2711, 1999.

Sih R, Morley JE, Kaiser FE, et al. Testosterone replacement in older
hypogonadal men: A 12 month randomized controlled trial. J Clin
Endocrinol Metab. 82: 1661–1667, 1997.

Snyder P. Effects of age on testicular function and consequences of testosterone treatment. J Clin Endocrinol Metab 86: 2369–2372, 2001.

Snyder PJ, Peachey H, Berlin JA, et al. Effects of testosterone replacement in
hypogonadal men. J Clin Endocrinol Metab 85: 2670–2677, 2000.

Snyder PJ, Peachey H, Hannoush P, et al. Effect of testosterone treatment on
body compostition and muscle strength in men over 65 years of age.
J. Clin Endocrinol Metab 84: 2647–2653, 1999.

Thompson P, Sadaniatz A, Cullinane E, Bodziony K, Catlin D. Left ventricu-
lar function is not impaired in weight-lifters who use anabolic steroids.
J Am Coll Cardiol 19: 278–282, 1992.

Wang C, Eyre DR, Clark R, Kleinberg D, Newman C, Iranmanesh A, et al.
Sublingual testosterone replacement improves muscle mass and strength,
decreases bone resorption, and increases bone formation markers in

hypogonadal men—a clinical research center study. J Clin Endocrinol Metab 81: 3654–2662, 1996.

Wang C, Swerdloff RS, Iranmanesh A, et al. Transdermal gel improves sexual function, mood, muscle strength, and body composition parameters in hypogonadal men. J Clin Endocrinol Metab 85: 2839–2853, 2000.

Wiebke A, Callies F, Koehler I, et al. Dehydroepiandrosterone supplementation in healthy men with an age-related decline of dehydroepiandrosterone secretion. J Clin Endocrinol Metab 86: 4686–4692, 2001.

Wiebke A, Haas J, Callies F, et al. Biotransformation of oral dehydroepiandrosterone in elderly men: Significant increase in circulating estrogen. J Clin Endocrinol Metab 84: 2170–2176, 1999.

Yen SS. Dehydroepiandrosterone sulfate and longevity: New clues for an old friend. Proc Natl Acad Sci USA 98: 8167–8169, 2001.

Chapter 15

Andriol advertisement in Asian Journal of Andrology. 3: 161–240, 2001.

Arver S, Dobs AS, Meikle AW, et al. Improvement in sexual function in testosterone deficient men treated for one year with a permeation enhanced testosterone transdermal system. J Urol 155: 1604–1608, 1999.

Bloom BS, Iannacona RC. Internet availability of prescription pharmaceuticals to the public. Ann Intern Med 830–383, 1999.

Erinoff L, Lin GC (Ed.). National Institute on Drug Abuse Research Monograph Series: Anabolic Steroid Abuse. U.S. Dept. of Health and Human Services, Washington DC, 1990.

Klatz R, Kahn C. Grow Young with HCG. Harper Perennial, New York, 1998.

Meikle AW, Arver S Dobs AS, et al. Pharmacokinetics and metabolism of a permeation-enhanced testosterone transdermal system in hypogonadal men: Influence of application site. J Clin Endocrinol Metab 81: 1832–1840, 1996.

Perls TT, Silver MH. Living to 100. Basic Books, New York, 1999.

Reidenberg MM, Conner BA. Counterfeit and substandard drugs. Clin Pharmacol Ther, 69: 189–193, 2001.

SmithKline Beecham Pharmaceuticals. Andropatch Testosterone Transdermal System, Summary of Product Characteristics. London, U.K. 1996.

Solvay Pharmaceuticals, Inc. AndroGel Summary of Product Characteristics. 2000.

Wagner JC. Abuse of drugs used to enhance athletic performance. Am J Hosp Pharm 46: 2760–2067, 1989.

Chapter 16

Anderson RA, Martin CW, Kung AWC, et al. 7-Alpha-methyl-19-nortestosterone maintains sexual behavior and mood in hypogonadal men. J Clin Endocrinol Metab 84: 35566–3562, 1999.

Anderson RA, and Wu FCW. Comparison between testosterone enanthate-induced azoospermia and oligospermia in a male contraceptive study. J Clin Endocrinol Metab 81: 896–901, 1996.

Kumar N, Small M, Sundaram K. 7-Alpha-methyl-19-nortestosterone (MENT®): An Ideal Androgen. The Population Council, New York, 2000.

Kumar N, Didolkar AK, Ladd A. Radioimmunoassay of 7-alpha-methyl-19-nortestosterone and investigation of its pharmacodynamics in animals. J Steroid Biochem Mol Biol 37: 587–591, 1990.

Kumar N, Didolkar AK, Monder C, et al. The biological activity of 7-alpha-methyl 19-nortestosterone is not amplified in the male reproductive tract as is that of testosterone. Endocrinology 130: 3677–3683, 1992.

LaMorte A, Kumar N, Bardin CW, Sundaram K. Aromatization of 7-alpha-methyl-19-nortestosterone by human placental microsomes in vitro. J Steroid Biochem Mol Biol 48: 287–304, 1994.

Population Council. Male Contraceptive Development: MENT®. Population Council, New York, 2002.

Population Council. MENT® Licensing Agreement Signed. Population Council, New York, 2000.

Sundaram K, Kumar N, Bardin CW. 7-Alpha-methyl-19-nortestosterone (MENT): The optimal androgen for male contraception. Ann Med 25: 199–205, 1993.

Sundaram K, Kumar N, Monder C, et al. Different patterns of metabolism determine the relative anabolic activity of 19-norandrogens. J Steroid Biochem Mol Biol 53: 253–257, 1995.

Suvisaari J, Moo-Young A, Juhakoski, A. et al. Pharmacokinetics of 7 alpha-methyl-19-nor-testosterone (MENT®) delivery using subdermal implants in healthy men. Contraception 60: 299–303, 1999.

Suvisaari J, Sundaram K, Noe G, et al. Pharmacokinetics and pharmacodynamics of 7-alpha-methyl-19-nortestosterone (MENT) after intramuscular administration in healthy men. Hum Reprod 12: 967–973, 1997.

Tenover JS. Effects of testosterone supplementation in the aging make. J Clin Endocrinol Metab 75: 1092–1097, 1992.

Winters SJ. Current status of testosterone replacement therapy in men. Arch Fam Med 8: 257–263, 1996.

Chapter 17

Bardin CW, Swerdloff RS, Santen RJ. Androgens: Risks and benefits. J Clin Endocrinol Metab 73: 4–7, 1991.

Barrett-Connor E, Khaw KT, Yen SS. A prospective study of dehydroepiandrosterone sulfate, mortality, and cardiovascular disease. N Eng J Med 315: 1519–1524, 1986.

Bulbrook, RD, Hayward JL, Spicer CC. Abnormal excretion of urinary steroids by women with early breast cancer. Lancet 2: 1238–1240, 1962.

Bagatell CJ, Bremner WJ. The effects of aging and testosterone on lipids and cardiovascular risk. J Clin Endocrinol Metab 83: 3440–3441, 1998.

Korenman SG. A pragmatic approach to androgen replacement in older men: Risks *vs* benefits. J Clin Endocrinol Metab 83: 3441–3443, 1998.

Medical Post. Male hormone supplements not bad for heart after all. April 21, 1998, vol. 34, no. 15.

Vermeulem A. Androgen replacement in the aging male—A critical evaluation. J Clin Endocrinol Metab 86: 2380–2390, 2001.

Wiebke A, Hass J, Callies F, et al. Biotransformation of oral dehydroepiandrosterone in elderly men: Significant increase in circulating estrogens. J Clin Endocrinol Metab 84: 2170–2176, 1999.

Chapter 18

Arlt W, Callies F, Koehler I, et al. Dehydroepiandrosterone supplementation in healthy men with an age-related decline in dehydroepiandrosterone secretion. J Clin Endocrinol Metab 86: 4686–4692, 2001.

Arlt W, Haas J, Callies F, et al. Biotransformation of oral dehydroepiandrosterone in elderly men: Significant increase in circulating estrogens. J Clin Endocrinol Metab 84: 2170–2176, 1999.

Barrett-Connor E, Kwah KT, Yen, SS, A prospective study of dehydroepiandrosterone sulfate, mortality, and cardiovascular disease. N Eng J Med 315: 1519–1524, 1986.

Broeder CE, Quidry J, Brittingham K, et al. The Andro Project: Physiological and hormonal influences of androstenedione supplementation in men 35 to 65 years old participating in a high-intensity resistance training program. *Arch Intern Med* 160: 3093–3104, 2000.

Brown GA, Vukovich MD, Sharp RL, et al. Effect of oral DHEA on serum testosterone and adaptations to resistance training in young men. J Appl Physiol 87: 2274–2283, 1999.

Brown, GA, Vukovich MD, Martini E, et al. Endocrine responses to chronic androstenedione intake in 30- to 56-year-old men. J Clin Endocrinol Metab 85: 4074–4080, 2000.

Bulbrook RD, Hayward JL, Spicer CC. Abnormal excretion of urinary steroids by women with early breast cancer. Lancet 2: 1238–1240, 1962.

Chass, M. Vantage Point. Slow Bonds to a walk? International Herald Tribune, April 6–7, 2002, p. 21.

Dean W, Fowkes SW. DHEA. *Smart Drug News*, October 15, 2, 1993.

Gen.com. AndroGen. Product description sheet. www.Gen.com, Feb. 11, 2000.

Justice R. Baseball studies Andro. *Washington Post*, February 9, 2000; p. D01.

Kahn AT, Halloran B. Dehydroepiandrosterone supplementation and bone turnover in middle-aged to elderly men. J Clin Endocrinol Metab 87: 1544–1549, 2002.

King DS, Sharp RL, Vukovich MD, et al. Effect of oral androstenedione on serum testosterone and adaptations to resistance training in young men: a randomized control trial. JAMA 281: 2043–2044, 1999.

King DS, et al. Effect of oral androstenediol on serum testosterone and adaptation to training in young men. JAMA 281: 2020–2028, 1999.

Kuhn C. Anabolic steroids. Recent Prog Horm Res 57: 411–434, 2002.

Kutscher EC, Lund BC, Perry PJ. Anabolic steroids: A review for the clinician. Sports Med. 32: 285–296. 2002.

Leder, BZ, Longcope C, Catlin DH, et al. Oral androstenedione administration and serum testosterone concentrations in young men. JAMA 283: 779–782, 2000.

Legrain S, Massien C, Baulieu EE, et al. Dehydroepiandrosterone replacement administration: Pharmacokinetic and pharmacodynamic studies in healthy elderly subjects. J Clin Endocrinol Metab. 85: 3208–3217, 2000.

Mahesh VG, Greenblatt RB. The in vivo conversion of dehydroepiandrosterone and androstenedione to testosterone in the human. Acta Endocrinol 41: 400–406, 1962.

Markel D, Kaplan N, Fishel M. The Andro Debate. Angelfire.com on the Internet, February 12, 2002.

Nagourney E. Consequences: Athletes, andro and trouble in the urine. *New York Times*, Science section: 1, November 28, 2000.

Orensreich N, Brind JH, Vogelman RA, Baldwin H. Long-term longitudinal measurements of plasma dehydroepiandrosterone sulfate in normal men. J Clin Endocrinol Metab 75: 1002–1004, 1992.

Parssinen M, Seppala T. Steroid use and long-term health risks in former athletes. Sports Med. 32: 83–94, 2002.

Rasmussen BB, Volpi E, Gore, DC, Wolfe RR. Androstenedione does not stimulate muscle protein anabolism in young health men. J Clin Endocrinol Metab 85: 55–59, 2000.

Schnirring L. Study raises doubts about claims for "Andro." The physician and sports medicine, Vol. 27, no. 8: August, 1999.

Sports Illustrated. Steroids in baseball (special report). May 28, 2002.

Trivedi DP, Khaw KT. Dehydroepiandrosterone sulfate and mortality in elderly men and women. J Clin Endocrinol Metab 86: 4171–4177, 2001.

USA Today. Steroids in sports. July 9, 2002.

Verducci, T. Steroids in baseball: The injury toll. *Time Magazine* June 3, 2002, p. 44.

Wallace MB, Lim J. Cutler A, Bucci, L. Effects of dehydroepiandrosterone vs androstenedione supplementation in men. Med Sci Sports Exerc 31: 1788–1792, 1999.

Weil A. Natural Health, Natural Medicine. Houghton Mifflin, Boston, 1998.

Williams, MRI, Ling SH, Dawood T, et al. Dehydroepiandrosterone inhibits human vascular smooth muscle cell proliferation independent of ARs and ERs. J Clin Endocrinol Metab 87: 176–181, 2002.

Woolston C. Androstenediol (Andro): Buyer Beware. A healthy me.com on the Internet. 2001.

Yen SSC. Dehydroepiandrosterone sulfate and longevity: New clues for an old friend. Proc Natl Acad Sci USA 98: 8167–8169, 2001.

Yesalis CE III. Medical, legal, and societal implications of androstenedione use. JAMA 281: 2043–2044, 1999.

Zorpette G. Andro angst. Sci Am 253: 16–25, 1998.

Chapter 19

Anderson RA, Martin CW, Kung AWC, et al. 7-alpha methyl 19 nor testosterone maintains sexual behavior and mood in hypogonadal men. J Clin Endocrinol Metab 84: 3559–3562, 1999.

Christiansen K, Kussman R. Sex hormones and cognitive function. Neuropsychobiology 18: 27–36, 1997.

Davidson, JM, Chen JJ, Crapo L, et al. Hormonal changes and sexual function in aging men. J Clin Endocrinol Metab 57: 71–77, 1983.

Ford WCL, North K, Taylor H, et al. Increasing paternal age is associated with delayed conception in a large population of fertile couples: Evidence for declining fecundity in older men. Hum Reprod 15:1703–1708, 2000.

Hajjar RR, Kaiser FE, Morley JE. Outcomes of long-term testosterone replacement in older hypogonadal males: a retrospective analysis. J Clin Endocrinol Metab 82: 3793–3796, 1997.

Johnson L, Petty CS, Neaves WB. Influence of age on sperm production and testicular weights in men. J Reprod Fertil 70: 211–218, 1984.

Johnson L, Zane RS, Petty CS, Neaves WB. Quantification of the human Sertoli cell population: its distribution, relation to germ cell number, and age-related decline. Biol Reprod 31: 785–795, 1984.

Kolata, G. Male hormone therapy popular but untested. *New York Times*, August 19, 2002, p. 1.

Korenman SG, Morley JE, Mooradian AD, et al. Secondary hypogonadism in older men: Its relation to impotence. J Clin Endocrinol Metab 71: 963–969, 1990.

Ly, LP, Jimenez M, Zhwuang, TN, Celermajer, et al. A double-blind, placebo-controlled, randomized clinical trial of transdermal dihydrotestosterone gel on muscular strength, mobility, and quality of life in older men with partial androgen deficiency. J Clin Endocrinol Metab 86: 4078–4088, 2001.

Morley JE. Testosterone. In: Contemporary Endocrinology: Endocrinology of Aging, Morley JE, van den Berg L. (Eds.). Humana Press, Totowa, NJ, 1999, 49–55.

Morley JE, Perry HM, Kaiser FE, et al. Effect of testosterone replacement therapy in old hypogonadal males. J Am Geriatr Soc 41: 149–152, 1993.

Neischlag E, Lammers U, Freishem CW, et al. Reproduction functions in young fathers and grandfathers. J Clin Endocrinol Metab 55: 676–681, 1982.

Paulson RJ, Milligran RC, Sokol, RZ. The lack of influence of age on male fertility. Am J Obstet Gynecol 184: 816–824, 2001.

Reiter WJ, Pycha A, Schatzl G, Gruber DB, Huber JC, Marberger M. Dehydroepiandrosterone in treatment of erectile dysfunction: A prospective double-blind randomized placebo-controlled study. Urology 53: 590–594, 1999.

Rowe JW, Kahn RL. Successful Aging. Pantheon Books, New York, 1998.

Schiavi RC, Schreiner-Engel P, White D, et al. The relationship between pituitary-gonadal function and sexual behavior in healthy aging men. Psychosom Med 53: 363–374. 1991.

Sih R, Morley JE, Kaiser FE, et al. Testosterone replacement in older hypogonadal men: A twelve month randomized controlled trial. J Clin Endocrinol Metab 82: 1661–1667, 1997.

Tenover JS. Effects of testosterone supplementation in the aging male. J Clin Endocrinol Metab. 76: 1092–1098, 1992.

Tenover JS. Male hormone replacement therapy including "andropause." Endocrinol Metab Clin N Am. 27: 969–987, 1998.

Wang C, Swerdloff RS, Iranmanesh A, and the Testosterone Gel Study Group. Transdermal testosterone gel improves sexual function, mood, muscle strength, and body composition parameters in hypogonadal men. J Clin Endcrinol Metab 85: 2839–2853, 2000.

Chapter 20

Almeida OP, Barclay L. Sex hormones and their impact on dementia and depression: A clinical perspective. Expert Opin Pharmacother 2: 527–535, 2001.

Anderson RA, Martin CW, Kung AWC, et al. 7-Alpha methyl 19 nor testosterone maintains sexual behavior and mood in hypogonadal men. J Clin Endocrinol Metab 84: 3559–3562, 1999.

Baber J, Bongers G, LeFevour A, et al. Androgens protect against apolipoprotein E-4 induced cognitive deficits. J Neurosci 22: 5204–5209, 2002.

Barrett-Connor E, Goodman-Gruen D, Patay B. Endogenous sex hormones and cognitive function in older men. J Clin Endocrinol Metab 84: 4681–3695, 1999.

Barrett-Connor E, Von Muhlen DG, Kritz-Silverstein D. Bioavailable testosterone and depressed mood in older men: The Rancho Bernardo Study. J Clin Endocrinol Metab 84: 573–575, 1999.

Cherrier MM, Asthana S, Plymate S, et al. Testosterone supplementation improves spatial and verbal memory in healthy older men. Neurology 57: 80–88, 2001.

Christiansen K, Kussman R. Sex hormones and cognitive function. Neuropsychobiology 18: 27–36, 1987.

Drew SV. Cognitive function after HRT. Lancet 357: 641, 2001.

Gouchie C, Kimura D. The relationship between testosterone levels and cognitive ability patterns. Psychoneurobiology 16: 323–334, 1991.

Hogervorst E, Lehmann DJ, Warden DR, et al. Apolipoprotein E epsilon 4 and testosterone interact in the risk of Alzheimer's disease in men. Int J Geriatr Psych 17: 938–940, 2002.

Hogervorst E, Williams J, Budge M, et al. Serum testosterone is lower in men with Alzheimer's disease. Neuroendocrinol Lett 22 (3): 163–816, 2001.

Janowski SC, Oviatt SH, Orwoll ES. Testosterone influences spatial cognition in older men. Behav Neurosci 108: 325–332, 1994.

Kenny AM, Bellantonio S, Gruman CA, et al. Effects of transdermal testosterone on cognitive function and health perception in older men with low bioavailable testosterone levels. J Gerontol A Biol Sci Med 57: M321–325, 2002.

Kolata G. Male hormone therapy popular but untested. New York Times, August 19, 2002, p. 1.

Ly LP, Jimenez M, Zhwuang TN, et al. A double-blind, placebo-controlled, randomized clinical trial of transdermal dihydrotestosterone gel on muscular strength, mobility, and quality of life in older men with partial androgen deficiency. J Clin Endocrinol Metab 86: 4078–4088, 2001.

Papasozomenos SCh, Shanavas A. Testosterone prevents the heat shock-induced overactivation of glycogen synthase kinase-3 beta but not of cyclin-dependent kinase-5 and c-Jun NH2–terminal kinase and concomitantly abolishes hyperphosphorylation of tau: Implications for Alzheimer's disease. Proc Natl Acad SCI USA 99: 1140–1145, 2002.

Wang C, Swerdloff RS, Iranmanesh A, et al. Transdermal testosterone gel improves sexual function, mood, muscle strength, and body composition parameters in hypogonadal men. J Clin Endocrinol Metab 85: 2839–2853, 2000.

Wolf OT, Kirschbaum C. Endogenous estradiol and testosterone are associated with cognitive performance in older women and men. Horm Behav 41: 259–266, 2002.

Yaffe K, Lui LY, Zmuda J, Cauley J. Sex hormones and cognitive function in older men. J Am Geriatr Soc 50: 707–712, 2002.

• • • Index

Antiandrogens, 104
Antiestrogens, 71–72
Antioxidants, 58, 62, 157
Aphrodisiac, 55, 157
Apoptosis, 41
Aromatase, 87, 157
Aromatization, 82
Arteriosclerosis, 81, 94, 158
Artificial insemination, 122–123
Aspirin, 62, 130
Assisted reproduction technology (ART), 44, 47–48
Astroglide, 66
Atherosclerosis, 34, 48, 94, 118, 158
Atresia, 3, 5, 6, 80, 158
Australia, 67
Ayurvedic medicine, 51, 158

Bardin, Wayne, 105
Baseball Player's Association, 116
Bazedoxifene, 75
Benign prostatic hypertrophy, (BPH), 110
Beta-amyloid. *See* Alzheimer's disease
Beta carotene, 62
Bioactive testosterone, 80
Bioethics, 47
Biologically active androgens, 83
Biphosphonates, 158
Black cohosh, 54, 55, 137
Blood-brain barrier, 130
Blue cohosh, 54
Body composition, 90
Bonds, Barry, 115
Bone density, 3, 13, 58, 60, 63, 72, 75, 87, 93, 105, 152
Bone remodeling, 27, 93, 140
Brazil, 61
Breast cancer, 19, 28, 29, 30, 31, 58, 71, 74
    antiestrogens for prevention of, 73
    environmental risk factors, 28
    genes for, 29
    HT as promoter of, 19, 30, 141–143
Breast enlargement in men, 87, 118
Breast feeding, duration of, 6
Breast tenderness, 51
Brigham and Women's Hospital, 33

Cache County study, 40
Calcium and vitamin D, 23, 51, 94
California Department of Health Services, 53
California study of sperm counts in men, 125
Cardiovascular disease, 57, 60, 74, 84
Cataract formation, 26
Central nervous system, 66
Chasteberry, 54, 56
China, 60
Chinese traditional medicine, 51
Chiropractic massage, 50
Cholesterol, 13, 34, 58, 72–73, 111, 121, 155
Circulation, 35
Climera, 17
Clitoris, 65
Clomiphene citrate, 71
Cognition, 126, 158
    effect of androgen decline on, 83
    neuropsychological tests, as measure of, 129
Colon cancer, 27, 36, 143–144
Columbia University, 39
Combi-Patch, 16–17
Contraception, 143
Controlled Substance Act of the U.S., 110
Cornell University, 28, 29
Coronary artery disease, 21, 33, 35
Corpus luteum, 10, 12, 157
Cost of new drug development, 74
Coumadin, 53, 56
Coutinho, Elsimar, 66
Crinone, 18
Cyproterone acetate, 104
Cytoplasmic transfer, 48–49

Damiana, 54
Dehydroepiandrosterone, 67, 86, 98, 119, 116–117, 154, 159
    manufacturer's recommended dose, 117
    production rate changes with aging, 119
    reported benefits for men, 86
    role in body's synthesis of testosterone, 86